STRATEGIC PLANNING FOR NURSES

Change Management in Health Care

Michele V. Sare, MSN, RN
Founder
Nurses for Nurses International
Missoula, Montana

LeAnn Ogilvie, MSN, RN, CCRN
Executive Member
Nurses for Nurses International
Missoula, Montana

JONES AND BARTLETT PUBLISHERS
Sudbury, Massachusetts
BOSTON   TORONTO   LONDON   SINGAPORE

World Headquarters
Jones and Bartlett Publishers
40 Tall Pine Drive
Sudbury, MA 01776
978-443-5000
info@jbpub.com
www.jbpub.com

Jones and Bartlett Publishers
Canada
6339 Ormindale Way
Mississauga, Ontario L5V 1J2
Canada

Jones and Bartlett Publishers
International
Barb House, Barb Mews
London W6 7PA
United Kingdom

Jones and Bartlett's books and products are available through most bookstores and online booksellers. To contact Jones and Bartlett Publishers directly, call 800-832-0034, fax 978-443-8000, or visit our website, www.jbpub.com.

Substantial discounts on bulk quantities of Jones and Bartlett's publications are available to corporations, professional associations, and other qualified organizations. For details and specific discount information, contact the special sales department at Jones and Bartlett via the above contact information or send an email to specialsales@jbpub.com.

The authors, editor, and publisher have made every effort to provide accurate information. However, they are not responsible for errors, omissions, or for any outcomes related to the use of the contents of this book and take no responsibility for the use of the products and procedures described. Treatments and side effects described in this book may not be applicable to all people; likewise, some people may require a dose or experience a side effect that is not described herein. Drugs and medical devices are discussed that may have limited availability controlled by the Food and Drug Administration (FDA) for use only in a research study or clinical trial. Research, clinical practice, and government regulations often change the accepted standard in this field. When consideration is being given to use of any drug in the clinical setting, the healthcare provider or reader is responsible for determining FDA status of the drug, reading the package insert, and reviewing prescribing information for the most up-to-date recommendations on dose, precautions, and contraindications, and determining the appropriate usage for the product. This is especially important in the case of drugs that are new or seldom used.

Production Credits

Publisher: Kevin Sullivan
Acquisitions Editor: Emily Ekle
Acquisitions Editor: Amy Sibley
Associate Editor: Patricia Donnelly
Editorial Assistant: Rachel Shuster
Associate Production Editor: Katie Spiegel
Marketing Manager: Rebecca Wasley

V.P., Manufacturing and Inventory Control: Therese Connell
Composition: Cape Cod Compositors, Inc.
Cover Design: Scott Moden
Cover Image: © Sgame/Dreamstime.com
Printing and Binding: Malloy, Inc.
Cover Printing: Malloy, Inc.

Library of Congress Cataloging-in-Publication Data
Sare, Michele V.
  Strategic planning for nurses : change management in health care / Michele V. Sare and LeAnn Ogilvie.
     p. ; cm.
  Includes bibliographical references and index.
  ISBN 978-0-7637-6617-7
  1. Strategic planning. 2. Nursing services—Administration. I. Ogilvie, LeAnn. II. Title.
  [DNLM: 1. Health Planning—methods. 2. Nursing Care—organization & administration. 3. Nursing—trends. 4. Organizational Innovation. WY 105 S244s 2010]
  RT89.S27 2010
  362.173—dc22
                                                                                      2009010233

6048

Printed in the United States of America
13 12 11 10 09   10 9 8 7 6 5 4 3 2 1

In loving memory of Michele's pragmatic, problem-solving engineer father, Del Sare, who built bridges, dams, roads, and undersea pipelines from the jungles of Borneo to the deserts of Afghanistan to the ice rocks of Greenland. He knew that in order to accomplish great feats, a clear plan and set of strategies were essential.

Contents

How to Use This Textbook

This book is divided into 3 parts with 11 chapters that lead the reader through the why's, how's, who's, and what's next of strategic planning applied specifically to nursing:

Part 1: Nursing and a New Frontier: The Need for Strategic Planning
Part 2: The Principles and Foundations of Strategic Planning
Part 3: Architects, Change Agents, and Communicators: Digging a Little Deeper

Each of the three parts can be studied independently; however, combined they clearly illustrate the purpose of this textbook, which is to teach the reader how to engage the strategic planning process to effect positive change in nursing today. The textbook explains the constructs of strategic planning, delivers in-depth instruction on the strategic planning process as it applies to nursing, and guides the reader to consider approaches and techniques to empower nursing through the utilization of proficient strategic planning.

This text can be used to augment leadership, management, or business courses, as a stand-alone course, or as a self-study textbook. All chapters begin with clear behavioral objects and contain self-directed learning assessments. A curriculum guide for educators is available through Jones and Bartlett Publishers. Please visit http://www.jbpub.com/nursing to download instructor resources.

Introduction

This book's goal is to strengthen nursing by offering a nurse-based perspective of key business skills. This text illustrates a new paradigm for nursing, but it teaches a way of thinking and practicing that has been adopted and ingrained in many other professional arenas, most specifically in the culture, domain, and sphere of influence of business and in the many realms that the concepts, skills, and explicit nature of business encompass. In any business-related book, Web site, conference, or other media product on topics from management styles to quality initiatives, for profit or not-for-profit "business" paradigms are the drivers. Nurses have stayed outside of the business playing field for too long.

Strategic Planning for Nurses: Change Management in Health Care builds insight and breaks boundaries that have historically hampered nursing's professional progression and power as a stakeholder in an ever-changing global business-based healthcare arena. This text offers specific skill and knowledge-based instruction on strategic planning concepts, trends, and issues that face the demographically and culturally diverse nursing workforce of the 21st century.

Nurses must learn to speak the language of business in order to overcome the pervasive sense of disempowerment that plagues the profession. Acquiring basic business skills and knowledge helps to increase autonomy, facilitate collaboration, and effect decision making within nursing's scope and domain. The intent of this book is to better prepare the nursing workforce to function, compete, and thrive in dynamic healthcare arenas and in the 21st century economy. A congruent intent is to augment and strengthen nursing knowledge and skill sets with competencies that have yet to be integrated into nursing education and practice across all levels—skills and knowledge that are fundamental to business, but have yet to be adopted as core competencies in nursing.

Nursing shortages, high turnover rates, chasms in quality of care, and cross-cultural disillusionment in nursing are results of disempowerment—a result of the chronic conundrum of a care-based professional model colliding with a healthcare marketplace, which wields authoritative control over care, which is based on a business model. Nurses must learn and understand universal and fundamental business practices to better relate, communicate, effect change, and assert and empower their professional product—care—in an industry that has a plethora of drivers. Nurses need sound basic business skills to shed the cloak of being "just a nurse" and take a stronger position in the boardroom, within organizations, and within political structures to strengthen the nursing profession.

Nurses at every level, from LPN to PhD, need clear business tools that are specific to the culture, needs, and environments where and how nursing practices. This book is the logical start into business for all nurses; the strategic planning process requires that values and visions be the starting point for all planning, change, and action.

Acknowledgments

In our collective 49 years as professional nurses, we have been enriched by and benefited from the humanity in our profession; nurse's aides, LPNs, RNs, and advanced practice nurses have influenced how we see our personal and professional lives. Student nurses have challenged us and helped us to grow. At the very heart of this book is our desire to strengthen nurses themselves. We are honored by and proud of the kind hearts and bright minds that choose the profession of care. It is your dedication, compassion, empathy, skill, and vast knowledge that drive us to want to improve the conditions of nursing. Thank you to every provider of care who has been a part of our journey.

Thank you to Michele's sister, Susan Hodges, who offered editing advice and helped us keep the mixed metaphors to a minimum. Peggy Stevens, Julie Serstad, Carrie Stensrud, and Cindy Jimmerson, all RN leaders, offered examples of how strategic planning has strengthened their professional practice. Many peers offered encouragement, reviewed ideas, and expressed the need for a book to help navigate the business arena—we would like to especially thank a nurse mentor extraordinaire, Karen Hill. Michele's son, Jesse, was the technical computer master who kept the process going, and LeAnn's family supported her long days and need for computer time. Thank you all!

Transforming our work into a book involved many people with remarkable skill and talent. We would like to thank the editorial and production staff at Jones and Bartlett Publishers, who patiently and kindly guided us through this project: Emily Ekle, Rachel Shuster, Katie Spiegel, Julie McLaughlin, and the rest of the team.

Michele V. Sare and LeAnn Ogilvie

Contributors

Cindy Jimmerson, RN
Lean Healthcare West
Bonner, Montana

Julie Serstad, MSN, RN
Director of Health Services, Missoula City-County Health Department
Missoula, Montana

Carrie Stensrud, BSN, RN, CCRN-CSC
Saint Patrick Health Sciences Center
Missoula, Montana

Peggy Stevens, BSN, RN
Lead Public Health Official
Mineral County, Montana

PART 1

Nursing and a New Frontier: The Need for Strategic Planning

Why Nursing Needs Strategic Planning: Professional Empowerment in the New Millennium

> *"In action be primitive; in foresight, a strategist."*
> —René Char, 1907–1988

Strategic planning is a terrific tool used in business everywhere to effect positive change; it is logical, timely, vital, empowering, and a really fun process. Strategic planning solves problems and establishes a wonderful framework to guide decision-making. Strategic planning truly is very helpful as a process tool that is useful at every level of nursing practice. Nurses understand the nursing process; think of strategic planning as an extended and expanded version of the nursing process that can be applied to projects, problems, and processes of every kind. In its truest form, strategic planning guides the future direction of a group or organization based on a thorough assessment of the present and some pretty spiffy forecasting of the future.

Strategic planning isn't without its pitfalls; perhaps you have been involved with or heard of a strategic plan that never got off the ground, or, if it did, it had a ridiculous crash landing; worse yet, the strategic plan was stuffed down your throat as a "you will do this." It's true that strategic planning needs many pieces; people need to do what they say they will do and, most important, to know what the plan actually is and believe in the plan. Have you ever planned a great family vacation, only to find out that your kids, spouse, or whoever thinks the vacation is horrible and complains all the way to the beach? Well, strategic planning can be like that, but it can also be the vacation of a lifetime that everyone absolutely loves!

Much of the literature on strategic planning is presented in the context of concepts that don't sound much like nursing—customer centers, marketing teams, and sales objectives. But the truth is that nurses work in a business land-scape, and your administration knows where the customer center is, who is on its marketing team, and what its sales objectives are. The territory of the busi-ness of health care is deeply immersed in competitive strategies—strategic plans that serve to secure your healthcare facility's market position. Being blissfully unaware of the business end of the stick has not served nursing well. We promise that strategic planning, as well as other "business skills," is quite fun and absolutely empowering, and acquiring some of these basic skills and knowledge will far better serve nurses and nursing.

CONNECTING NURSING TO STRATEGIC PLANNING

Strategic Planning for Nurses: Change Management in Health Care respects the culture, practice, and domain of nursing by applying strategic planning principles to nursing itself. It is not a cookie-cutter model of strategic planning imposed on nursing; this text is a compilation of principles that are aligned with the realities and culture of the nursing profession and a deep knowledge of the people who nurse.

One of the clearest and most empowering revelations has been to under-stand how "everyone else" sees their work and conducts their business, and how nursing is a part of a much bigger picture—a picture that resides within the realm of business. Health care is a business.

We were the ones who said, "Business and health care don't mix." We still deeply question the ethic of profiting from another's misfortune, and we do not abide by the philosophies that pit "consumers" against "manufacturers of care"; some of our current healthcare paradigms are inhuman. Until recently, many hospital mission statements clearly stated that their *primary* purpose was to increase shareholder wealth. OK, care has come into conflict with the "busi-ness" powers that are running the show. Standing on a soapbox and declaring foul will not change anything; that is victim thinking. Nursing needs to join in the business of health care in order to leverage influence, empower the profession, and improve care.

All nurses need to understand how to effectively survive and thrive with and within a business model while asserting and maintaining care excellence. It is time for nursing to remove the very real ceiling that encloses and stifles nursing. It is no glass ceiling; it is a ceiling constructed of a web of conflicting paradigms: shareholder wealth versus care excellence, market position versus care excellence, and administrative industrial paradigms versus care paradigms. If we are going to address workforce development, we must address those issues that undermine the strength and health of the profession. If we are to discuss "linkages," we must connect real-world need with education and practice that extends beyond what has "always been done." Health care is a business. Nurses work in a business. All nurses need business skills.

Nursing is a giant organization; this is what organizations do—they learn and refine skills to work more efficiently and to work together more effectively toward a shared vision. Perhaps the best (unintentional) endorsement for a book about strategic planning for nurses comes from the motto of the World Health Organization (WHO) for its Nursing and Midwifery program: "Thinking strategically, acting globally!" (2005).

YEAH, WE'VE HEARD—NURSING IS IN CRISIS

Is the job fundamentally flawed, or is it something else that has boardrooms all abuzz about this "crisis"? There is something about being told you are ill that has a way of making you feel ill. There is something about being told you have a problem that makes the problem feel "bigger." There is something about focusing on a problem that makes it feel like it may be hopeless, or at least hugely difficult to solve. Solutions make people feel better. Strategic planning and related business skills make a wonderful set of nursing process tools that can be applied to the profession to empower nurses. Instead of focusing on the ills, strategic planning and its related tools can remove that sense of icky helplessness.

Have you ever been around fellow staff in the break room who expound on all sorts of problems, with no shortage of examples? Those who sought a little reprieve from the challenges of the day leave the break room with a bigger burden and no rejuvenation to empower their work for the remainder of their shift. It isn't just in the break rooms; the dialogue is everywhere—in nursing journals, medical journals, the WHO's media, conference rooms, and newspapers; on television; in the U.S. Department of Public Health and Human Service's (DPHHS) media; and from the National League for Nursing (NLN,

2005, 2008) and the American Nurses Association (ANA, 1991). Politicians use the topic as a campaign platform. Is there anyone who does not know that "nursing is in crisis"?

Just in case you haven't gotten in on the wave of the "whatever are we to do?" hoopla of the past two decades, here's a little overview of the dilemma:

- The average age of nurses in 2000 was 44.5 years (Center for Nursing Advocacy, 2008).
- If current trends continue, the average age will reach 50 years by 2020 (Center for Nursing Advocacy, 2008).
- A total of 20–35% of nurses working in hospitals and nursing centers are not satisfied with their jobs (Biviano, 2003, slide 1).
- The United States is projected to have a shortfall of 808,416 nurses by 2020 (Health Resources and Services Administration [HRSA], 2002).
- The shortage is purported to reach 29% by 2020 in the United States (Biviano, 2003, slide 2).
- Many nursing job satisfaction polls point to three key variables that impact why nurses do not stay in nursing: lack of autonomy, poor or no collaboration in decision-making, and lack of control over the nurse's domain: care (Huff, 1997).
- There are 14,465,439 nurses worldwide, with a shortage of 43 million nurses in countries that need nursing the most (WHO, 2005); the shortage is an international problem.
- "The global profile . . . shows that there are more than 59 million health workers in the world, distributed unequally between and within countries. They are found predominantly in richer areas where health needs are less severe. Their numbers remain woefully insufficient to meet health needs, with the total shortage being in the order of 4.3 million workers" (WHO, 2006, p. 15).
- Nursing school admissions are hindered because of too few nursing faculty.
- Nursing retention rates are poor: 12–15% attrition (Doiron & Jones, 2006).
- A total of 31% of facilities in three states were not staffing at minimum (RN) staffing threshold levels (Government Accounting Office [GAO], 2001).
- Demographic forces are widening the gap between those needing care and those receiving care (GAO, 2001).
- "[There is] no end in sight for the nursing shortage" (Runy, 2005, p. 1).
- "Virtually all Americans will require nursing care at some time in their lives" (University-Wide Health Sciences Committee, 2004, p. 1).

Well, there you have it—a crisis! The literature abounds on the many tacks and methodologies that will address and solve the conundrum called the nursing crisis.

In 2005, the Nursing Organizations Alliance (Runy, 2005) set out nine principles to help curb the high rate of nursing attrition (Table 1-1). These principles are a wonderful start, but a very key player in this paradigm is missing; all of these solutions depend on "others" to solve the nursing crisis and flow from a top-down decision-making system. Most of the solutions are coming from "on high": administrators, human resource departments, politicians, regulatory and advisory agencies, academia, and managers and leaders in organizations and disciplines that have a stake in nursing (such as insurance companies).

Now is the time for grassroots change in nursing. Our leaders of tomorrow must come from the infallible congregation of nursing and need not be ensconced in academic institutions or in the hallways of administration. Nurses must understand basic principles of business to be a part of the solutions; understanding the strategic planning process is a very good starting point.

BENCHMARKS, COMPETENCIES, LINKAGES, AND EXCELLENCE: WE NEED A PLAN!

How long have you been in nursing? If you are a nursing learner, how long have you been around the healthcare industry? Have you seen any changes—new medications, new diseases, scary diseases, environmental threats that didn't exist a few years ago, new human threats like bioterrorism, and new weapons of mass destruction? How about new degrees or certifications? Do you know

---

Table 1-1   The Nursing Organizations Alliance's Nine Principles

1. Respectful collegial communication and behavior (no yelling doctors?)
2. Communication-rich culture
3. A culture of accountability (everyone—no blaming)
4. Presence of adequate numbers of qualified nurses (with work and home [in balance])
5. Presence of expert, credible, visible leadership
6. Shared decision-making at all levels
7. Encouragement of professional practice and growth and development
8. Recognition of the value of nursing's contribution
9. Recognition of nurses for their meaningful contribution to the practice

Source: Runy, 2005, pp. 1–2.

what all of that alphabet soup is at the end of your supervisor's name tag? Is your uniform different? Is that another new electronic medical record? Who bought that new IV pump that has more alarms than all the fire departments in New York City? What about all the information technology (IT) everything? Is that another new administrator? Did they change the mission statement again? "Nurse leader," she couldn't find her way in a well-lit preschool! How many classes do I need to take? What do you mean, that isn't how we do this anymore? I have to cover whose shift for how many hours, and you want me to attend how many meetings without pay? Sounds familiar doesn't it? It is just a glimpse of what an average day for a nurse might hold, regardless of the work setting.

The world of health care, the world of nursing, and the world of finance are changing. Today's global environment and the world of tomorrow have one indisputable constant: change. With all the variables that affect and sway nurses and nursing, change is omnipresent. But wait, there's more: chasms, errors, shortages, dissatisfaction, litigation, "consumer confidence," consumer satisfaction. At the end of the day, with a swirling culture of change and drivers, what really matters is client outcomes. We aren't doing very well with those, because too many interests are driving and fragmenting care!

With change at the speed of thought, nursing's stakeholders have proposed many solutions. These solutions are coming from "drivers" in packages called things like benchmarks and dashboards, evidenced-based nursing, competencies and linkages, Magnet Status, quality improvement initiatives, and performance excellence in practice.

To ensure understanding of what is meant by these key terms and forces of nursing practice, let's define the who, what, where, when, and how.

Drivers (forces). A driver is a force that operates and directs. We all know what it means to drive a car; we are at the controls, making all the decisions—turn left, turn right, stop, go backward. There are so many drivers in nursing that the profession sometimes hasn't got a clue about which direction it is headed—and some of the drivers are inexperienced, autocratic, or clueless about care. Drivers of nursing include supervisors, administration, licensing bodies, regulatory agencies, governing bodies, associations, organizations, political bodies, legal entities, nursing's hierarchy, and, above all, the client, patient, resident, and consumer. (One potentially key driver hasn't been heard from in an organized articulate voice: the nurse—not the entities "representing" the nurse, but the nurse herself.)

Benchmarks. A benchmark is a standard. The word *benchmark* is an engineering term used to identify a fixed point from which all other measurements are made. In the 1970s, benchmarking became a "systematic process of searching for best practices, innovative ideas and highly effective operating procedures that lead to superior performance" (Blakeman, 2002, p. 1). Benchmarking in nursing is sometimes referred to as "best practices" or "evidence-based practice"; it is the best of what we know at the time. Benchmarks change as new knowledge is discovered, and as you can imagine, there are hundreds of benchmarks for every area of practice

Dashboards. Dashboards are scorecards that keep track of where something is going and how it is doing; we think of it as an instrument panel of a vehicle. In 1846, *dash board* (two words) referred to a leather apron or a wooden board mounted on a horse-drawn carriage to prevent mud and yuck from being splashed on the travelers. Today, a dashboard (one word) is a grading, measurement, and tracking tool in business (kind of keeping track of the muck?).

Evidence-based nursing. This one is pretty easy; nurses don't do "what has always been done." Practice is based on the best information available at the time. For example, we used to think that everyone should stay in bed a good long time. We know today of the hazards of immobility. Nurses plan their care based on the best evidence. Another way to say it is "best practices."

Competency. Competency means ability or legal capacity. The term *competency* has been around as an evaluation tool since the 1960s, when a Harvard psychologist, David McClelland, developed a model to measure job performance. It wasn't until the 1990s that his ideas caught on. "Competencies" are a relatively new tool for management systems, and it is a concept that is gathering steam in the world of business. The ANA and the NLN have embraced the idea of basing performance measurement on competence criteria. There is even talk that a new pay scale model, "pay for performance," will be on nursing's horizon.

Linkages. Linkages involve linking one thing to another. Linkages in nursing refer to the links between education and practice, between nursing care and patient outcomes, and between the nursing process and outcomes. The Council on Linkages seeks to tie education to public health practice, and the North American Nursing Diagnosis Association to outcomes—the list goes on. Linkage is about alignment.

Magnet Status. The nursing shortage spawned the concept of attracting nurses—like a magnet—to hospitals that are wonderful to work at. The American Nurses Credentialing Center (2009) of the ANA created 14 criteria that would grant Magnet Status. Their credo for the creation of this gold standard of a "best place for nurses to work" (and therefore excellent patient care and outcomes) is called "magnetism."

Quality improvement initiatives. Total quality improvement (TQI), quality indicators (QIs), continuous quality improvement (CQI), and quality assessment (QA) are all terms for processes that seek to assure quality. These management tools come directly from the domain of business—how to make a better light bulb, a better cookie cutter, a better anything, in less time, at a lower cost, and using fewer resources. TQI and CQI are processes that seek to streamline and make optimally effective the use of all resources (human, time, money, materials, and transportation resources; facilities and operation expenses and skills; and talents and knowledge).

Excellence. Excellence is "outstanding quality" ("excellence," *Oxford Desk Dictionary,* 1995). *Excellence* is a vague term that is hard to quantify in and of itself; excellence in nursing is measured by benchmarks, evidence-based practice, and QIs such as outcomes. There are "centers of excellence" in every discipline; some are self-named, and some earned the title. An example in nursing is Magnet Status.

With so many drivers at the helm of nursing and so many ways to assess a nurse, it is vital for every nurse to be a part of the decision-making process. Otherwise, nurses (and nursing) will continue to feel as though they are dancing in step to an organ-grinder's tune. Nurses must join organizations that seek to represent the profession, but if all that is done is the paying of dues, the voice is not from the nurse; the voice is from those determining nursing's direction. Nursing has some wonderfully effective organizations, but members need clear skills to participate in any organizational process (alias: business process).

A WORD ABOUT DISEMPOWERMENT

Disempowerment, the most pervasive ill in nursing, is defined as taking away ability and removing authority. A chief complaint of nurses is a lack of autonomy (self-governance). It is a tangled web—so many drivers, so many puppeteers pulling on the strings of nursing. Not every nurse can sit at the boardroom table, but every nurse can learn how to effectively, efficiently, and intelligently work with and within the drivers of care.

To heal, nurses must learn new skills, new paradigms, and new ways of thinking about the vocation (industrial age) and the profession (knowledge age) of nursing. Both are necessary, both define nursing, and both are integral to healing us and launching us out of "crisis" status. Have you ever known anyone or anything that could be completely healed by others' Band Aids? Nurses well know that clients must want to get well and take control of their own health before they will quit smoking, lose weight, start exercising, or do anything else necessary to achieve health and well-being. Professions are no different: Disempowerment is at the heart of the nursing crisis. Empowerment then, is the only cure for the nursing crisis.

Empowerment is not solely about achieving competence within scope of practice; empowerment flows from the ability to effect positive change based on that scope of competence. For all nurses, the ultimate benefit of learning about the skills, knowledge, and processes of business is a strengthened position in the boardroom, a clearer voice in decision-making, and a more powerful voice as a client, consumer, patient, or resident advocate. With 14,465,439 nurses worldwide (WHO, 2005), nursing has the potential to be a very powerful voice, a voice that has not been well heard within nursing or by health care's stakeholders. An understanding of the principles of strategic planning is a vital first step to empowering the individual nurse and the vocational–professional continuum of nursing. The acquisition of these skills and knowledge sets is cardinal, timely, and essential to the professional health of nurses and nursing. We need a plan, we need to know how a plan works, and we need to be a part of the planning process!

NURSING'S DRIVERS: STANDARDS, GUIDELINES, AND ETHICS: THE BAR IS SET—IT'S PRETTY HIGH—HOW DO WE REACH IT?

We need to hear it one more time: It is important for all nurses to understand who and what the drivers of nursing are. Those drivers are making decisions that impact your work, your license, and, many times, your future in nursing. The ability to exert control over care should be the domain of nursing; the providers' domain is medical controls, physical therapy's control is a return to activity, respiratory therapy improves airways, and nurses care and provide care. It seems pretty straightforward, but with so many different interests and "cooks stirring the healthcare pot"—each trying to gain or maintain control over its piece of the healthcare pie and the healthcare dollar—the individual professional interests get diluted. Those professions that do not participate in the decision-making processes get the short end of the stick. There are a plethora of ways to "nurse"—from long-term care, to ICU, to school nursing and occupational health, to trauma care—and each subgroup of nursing has its own set of unique drivers.

Nursing has been feeling the ramifications of having to barter with that short stick, really, since Florence Nightingale's times. Did you know that the 37 nurses who went to serve in the Crimean War were not wanted? The "Lady of the Lamp" came about because the doctors would not allow the nurses around when they were working; the nurses could only work at night.

And to top it all off, there are many governing and regulatory bodies that exert some form of control over nursing. Sometimes, as the saying goes, if you don't know where you're going, someone will probably take you there. Unfortunately, this is a huge contributing factor to nurses' sense of lacking autonomy. Have you ever felt as though an administrator was leading nursing off on a wild goose chase? Perhaps you've even had a director of nursing who lost his or her way in care and was off on some paradigm that was in direct opposition to the science and theory of care, but you were not the one with "power" to sway the tide. There are nurses who, sad to admit, are so caught up in some form of angst or tangent that they are not even close to the core of nursing care. They have lost sight of the values and vision that first led them to the profession.

PROFESSION: REQUIRING SPECIALIZED AND ADVANCED TRAINING AND INTELLECTUAL ABILITY

The boards of nursing and various state agencies are responsible for the testing and licensure process. The National Council of State Boards of Nursing (NCSBN; state membership is optional) advises state boards and develops the NCLEX for both registered nurses (RNs) and practical nurses (PNs). The ANA advises these boards through their state affiliates by distributing their standards, guidelines, and ethics for nurses. The NLN sets the standards for nursing education. Both the ANA and the NLN influence the NCSBN and the state boards of nursing.

There are also regulatory bodies of nursing for almost every specialty area. In addition to specialty areas, there are subspecialty areas with unique regulatory and advisory organizations that set standards, guidelines, and ethics. Nurse practitioners (NPs) have organizations for the general field of advanced practice (AP), but there are also organizational aggregates for the subspecialties of AP and NP—for example, the American Academy of Nurse Practitioners and the American Association of Nurse Anesthetists. In a simple online search, I located more than 105 nursing organizations—that is a lot of nursing stakeholders with distinct agendas! If it isn't yet apparent to you, this alone should highlight the essential need for nursing to master business skills as a cardinal tool to keep the nursing profession speaking the same harmonious language.

NURSING IS A SCIENCE: SCIENCE IS BASED ON RESEARCH

Research is the order of the day. Nursing is a professional science and, as such, it must be founded on scientific reason and principles. Benchmarks, evidence-based practice, and excellence flow from the ongoing efforts of nursing research conducted through the DPHHS (the "mother" of all federal and state health programs and initiatives) and all the bodies within DPHHS: the Centers for Disease Control and Prevention, the National Institute of Nursing Research (NINR), and the Healthy People initiatives (to mention just a few) that drive funding and legislative thrust. Research also flows from academia, where many faculty cannot secure tenure unless they have conducted publishable research. Some research comes from the private sector, such as through foundations and grant efforts. Some research comes from nonnursing entities, like drug companies, and some comes from other healthcare entities, such as physical therapy or medicine.

Nursing will never be static. Research, by its very nature, continues to seek the best consistent results for all. At the very least, every nurse needs to strategically plan his or her professional development and portfolio just to keep up with research. It is also a good idea for all nurses to know where they want to go professionally and to know how to strategically position themselves within the profession, which will in turn help the profession to be strategically positioned. Change in nursing can feel like a swarm of stinging angry bees. With the right tools and, you guessed it, strategies, nurses need not get stung by the ongoing change and moving targets of benchmarks and best practices. A little strategic planning can reveal the path for the individual nurse and the nursing profession.

CHASMS—NURSING'S CHALLENGES FOR THE 21ST CENTURY: SERIOUS PROBLEMS THAT NEED CLEAR AND EFFECTIVE SOLUTIONS

We've reviewed some of the challenges facing nursing—those elements that inscribe the profession like a giant scarlet letter—earlier in this chapter: CRISIS. The Institute of Medicine (IOM) is a companion agency to three other agencies under the umbrella of the National Academies (created in 1863 by President Lincoln) to advise the government on matters of science and technology. Though not a government agency, the work of the IOM is directed by DPHHS and other governmental interests, and its work carries a great deal of clout with all healthcare stakeholders. Since the 1990s, the IOM has published several documents that bespeak the agony of today's healthcare system and the many chasms of care: CRISIS.

The IOM has not merely laid out the problem; its many publications offer solutions to the challenges. The IOM's multiple texts are edited by a multitude of professionals and experts. It is beyond the scope of this text to summarize all of the findings and proposed solutions; the only appropriate summary that can be offered is to implore the reader to access these works and to think deeply about their ramifications and implications. Please visit http://www.iom.edu/?id=7468 to view publications from the IOM since 1970. I think you'll be fascinated and will clearly see why nursing needs strategic planning!

THE IOM HAS A PRETTY CLEAR VISION—DO NURSES SEE IT TOO?

> *"The trouble with our times is that the future isn't what it used to be."*
> —Paul Valéry, 1871–1945

The broad swath of necessary change in the health care of the 21st century is universally evident. The world is connected in ways that were never imagined just 20 years ago, and it will be connected in the future in ways that are yet unknown. There are strategists, however, who are thinking about and planning for the changes. These strategists reside at places like the DPPHS, the IOM, and the NINR.

At the beginning of the millennium, we had hardly heard of "homeland security," and now almost every healthcare initiative is affected by concepts that did not hit our radar until 2001: bioterrorism, weapons of mass destruction, SARS, pandemic flu, and microbial resistance to what we thought were infallible antibiotics. There are those think-tankers who are helping to lead change, but too often, nursing has been in the position of reacting and not being the "think-tankee." As a nurse, what do you see for the next 5, 10, and 20 years for yourself and for the profession of nursing? Do you know what the IOM, the DPHHS, and the NINR see?

The DPHHS has given us a wonderful compendium of information that speaks to the strategic plan for America's entire healthcare system through Healthy People 2010. This information can be accessed at http://www.healthy people.gov. The National Association of City and County Health Officials held its national conference in conjunction with the Association of State and Territorial Health Officials in fall 2008. The theme for that conference was "Becoming the Healthiest Nation in a Healthier World" (http://www.naccho.org/ conferences). *Crossing the Quality Chasm: A New Health System for the 21st Century* "makes an urgent call for fundamental change to close the quality gap, recommends a redesign of the American health care system, and provides overarching principles for specific direction for policymakers, health care leaders, clinicians, regulators, purchasers, and others" (IOM, 2001). Do you know how to participate in these enterprise initiatives? Do you know how nursing was or was not involved in the creation of these concepts and mandates? Do you have the tools to be a participant?

The NINR has a strategic plan to promote health and prevent disease, to improve quality of life, to eliminate health disparities, and to set directions for end-of-life research (please see http://www.ninr.nih.gov/AboutNINR/ NINRMissionandStrategicPlan). How do you see yourself as a part of these strategies? How do "everyday" nurses join in these initiatives, these calls to action?

This is just a sampling of the strategic planning that is going on all around the profession of nursing. The facility where you work has a strategic plan. The board of directors has a strategic plan. The owners or stockholders have a strategic plan. Do you? Do you know how to join a team that is set to engage in strategic planning? Will you be able to engage the process effectively and efficiently? Most nurses cannot; we have never been asked to consider competencies that are not based on nursing science. If nursing is to shed the cloak of disempowerment, it must embrace the paradigms of business and the many magnificent tools of a business trade, and nurses must see themselves as members of the venture of health care.

We have cast a wide net to think about the drivers of nursing and the truth of constant change. We didn't talk about the patient, the consumer, or the resident, the ultimate drivers and change agents. The world's 15 million nurses have been charged with a remarkable duty: care for the world. With the plethora of conditions, environments, regulations, barriers, and drivers of care, nursing and nurses need sound tools of empowerment. Strategic planning is cool tool one.

Chapter 2 will take a look at the healthcare habitat and the new age of the knowledge worker. And, surprise! We will discover more ways that nursing will benefit from the ability to anticipate the future and from knowing how to be an instrument of change.

REVIEW QUESTIONS

1. How has terrorism impacted and changed the nursing profession?
2. Describe the differences between the terms *benchmarking, dashboard, evidence-based*, and *competency.*
3. What does it mean to be a "driver"?
4. What are the nine principles that the Nursing Organizations Alliance identified in 2005 to curb nursing attrition?
5. What is the difference between quality improvement initiatives and excellence?
6. What role does strategic planning play in the relationship between nurses and scientific research?

REFERENCES

American Nurses Credentialing Center (ANCC). (2009). Magnet Recognition Program®. Retrieved June 1, 2009, from http://www.nursecredentialing.org/Magnet.aspx

Biviano, M. (2003, April 23). The nursing crisis: Improving job satisfaction and quality of care. *Agency for Healthcare Research and Quality, National Center for Health Workforce Analysis*. Retrieved April 6, 2009, from http://www.ahrq.gov/news/ulp/workforctel/sess1/bivianotxt.htm

Blakeman, J. (June, 2002). *Benchmarking: Definitions and overview.* Retrieved April 6, 2009, from http://www.uwm.edu/Dept/CUTS/bench/bm-desc.htm

Center for Nursing Advocacy. (2008, January). *How many nurses are there? And other facts.* Retrieved April 5, 2009, from http://www.nursingadvocacy.org/rn_facts.html

Doiron, D., & Jones, G. (2006). Nurses' retention and hospital characteristics in New South Wales. *Economic Record, 82*(256), 11–29.

Excellence. (1995). In *Oxford Desk Dictionary American Edition.* New York: Oxford University Press.

Government Accounting Office (GAO). (2001, May 17). *Nursing workforce recruitment and retention of nurses and nurse aids is a growing concern.* Retrieved April 6, 2009, from http://www.gao.gov/new.items/d01750t.pdf

Health Resources and Services Administration (HRSA). (2002, July). *Projected supply, demand, and shortages of registered nurses: 2000–2020.* Retrieved April 6, 2009, from http://www.ahca.org/research/rnsupply_demand.pdf

Huff, C. (1997, October 23). Job satisfaction: Why your job isn't a bowl of cherries. *Nurseweek/Healthweek.* Retrieved April 6, 2009, from http://www.nurseweek.com/features/97-10/jobsatis.html

Institute of Medicine (IOM). (2001). *Crossing the quality chasm: A new health system for the 21st century.* Washington, DC: National Academies Press.

National League for Nursing (NLN). (2005, May 9). *Position statements.* Retrieved April 6, 2009, from http://www.nln.org/aboutnln/PositionStatements/index.htm

National League for Nursing (NLN). (2008). *Mission and goals.* Retrieved April 6, 2009, from http://www.nln.org/aboutnln/ourmission.htm

Runy, L. A. (2005). Nurse retention. *Hospitals & Health Networks.* Retrieved April 6, 2009, from http://www.hhnmag.com/hhnmag_app/jsp/articledisplay.jsp?dcrpath=HHNMAG/Article/data/11NOV2008/0811HHN_FEA_Gatefold&domain=HHNMAG

University-Wide Health Sciences Committee. (2004). *Nursing education and the University of California.* Retrieved April 6, 2009, from http://www.ucop.edu/hss/documents/nursing.pdf

World Health Organization (WHO). (2005). *The nursing and midwifery programme at WHO.* Retrieved April 6, 2009, from http://www.who.int/hrh/nursing_programme/en

World Health Organization (WHO). (2006). *Working together for health: The World Report 2006.* Retrieved April 6, 2009, from http://www.who.int/whr/2006/whr06_en.pdf

The Healthcare Habitat: The Evolving Professional Home of Nursing

——————— **OBJECTIVES** ———————

1. Describe how trends in nursing care (pay for performance, competency models, Magnet Status) impact the nursing profession.
2. Explain the relationship between the industry-age nurse and the knowledge-age nurse.
3. Identify and discuss the term *denursification*.
4. Discuss the origin and impact of quality control on health care.
5. Explore the importance of professional purpose through an exploration of your role in nursing's future.
6. Review the strategic plans of the Institute of Medicine, the World Health Organization, and the International Council of Nurses.
7. Review the future need for nurses and the financial impact of health care in the United States and globally.

The industrial age is fading over the horizon in many corners of business, the world economy, and the work environment of the 21st century. The work world is now connected in ways that most never imagined; it has been coined the "new global frontier." This shifting paradigm has many drivers that will continue to change the way work is done as well as who completes the work and where. Nursing must be a part of, and a driver of, this universal wave of change or become obsolete.

What does a changing healthcare environment, or habitat, have to do with strategic planning? Think about how care environments have changed. Does your facility still have a med-room, or is there a computer-based medication dispensing system? The first intensive care units (ICUs) came into being in the

1950s, but coronary care units (CCUs) were not developed until the 1960s. The ICUs and CCUs of today look nothing like those of the 1980s, and burn units are now extraordinarily specialized. Remember the isolation paraphernalia that used to reside outside an isolation room, with so many colors and types of signage? Thank goodness night nurses do not have to make the soap-suds enema solution any more! The healthcare environment—nursing habitat—has changed dramatically from wards and metal bedpans to modular units and portable X-rays.

As we move squarely into the 21st century, we can anticipate even greater changes in health care. One such shift has already occurred, wherein stand-alone surgery centers have replaced much of the surgical care previously provided under a hospital's structure. Healthcare "boutiques" and concierge medicine (also called "executive health care" and "platinum practices"— healthcare premiums paid as a retainer for exclusive health care) have cropped up in affluent neighborhoods. Telemedicine, telehealth, and telenursing are changing nursing's habitat. How about those electronic medical records (EMRs) and the proliferation of documentation changes; have they changed the nursing environment with networked computer terminals in every room? Some healthcare forecasters see the role of traditional hospitals fading from the scene and being replaced by newly designed community-based care.

With the majority of healthcare dollars being spent on acute care, payers of care (such as insurance companies) are desperate to cut expenditures and curb the need for acute care payments. (Ironically, disease prevention and health promotion efforts receive the fewest healthcare dollars.) In 2007, the United States spent a projected $2.26 trillion on health care, or $7,439 per person, and this figure is expected to increase by 6.7% annually—higher than the overall growth rate in the economy (4.9%) and general inflation (2.4%) (Centers for Medicare & Medicaid Services [CMS], 2008). Americans spend more per capita (for each person) and as a larger portion (16%) of the gross domestic product (GDP; values of all goods and services produced in a country in 1 year) than any other country (CMS, 2008). As the largest U.S. industry, health care employed over 14 million people in 2006 (2.5 million were registered nurses [RNs]; 59% of all hospital workers are RNs) and accounts for 7 of the 20 fastest growing occupations (Bureau of Labor Statistics [BLS], 2008a). Health care will generate 3 million new wage and salary jobs between 2006 and 2016, with nursing, including licensed practical nursing, as one of the occupations that that will continue to generate new jobs. The BLS predicts that the need for new RNs will be 587,000 (23% growth), and the need for licensed practical nurses (LPNs) will grow by 14% (or 105,000; BLS, 2008b). For both RNs and

LPNs in the United States, this projected growth rate is faster than in any other industry (BLS, 2008c).

Did you know what Homeland Security and the Federal Emergency Management Agency (FEMA) were 10 years ago? Have you noticed how antibiotic-resistant microbial strains have driven nursing practice? Until recently, *bioterrorism* was not a word that spell-checkers recognized. *Globalization* was a term that referred primarily to the domain of economics and financial and/or political entities such as the World Bank.

This is just the tip of the iceberg of the global healthcare environment; nursing's habitat has changed and will continue to change. One universal change that is occurring across all business entities is the shift from the industrial age to the knowledge age. The shift from the industrial age in many corners of business, the world economy, and the work environment of the 21st century has created new work possibilities. Understanding these influences is fundamental to leading change, and strategic planning is fundamental to participating in and effecting positive change in the healthcare habitat of the 21st century.

DAWNING OF A "NEW AGE": THE KNOWLEDGE WORKER

Professional disciplines everywhere have acknowledged, and are evolving in response to, the information age and the age of the knowledge worker. Nursing grew up in the industrial age, just like the auto industry, in which skills and technique were the arms of the "brains behind the machine." An engineer, a doctor, or a line manager decided on the need and the plan, and the muscle-reflexor on the assembly line, or in the sanatorium hall (clad in white and careful not to let those ankles show), would carry out the tasks of putting the plan together. The industrial workers usually didn't get to see the whole plan; their task was just to know where bolt A attached to locknut B, or when to administer enema A to patient B.

With technology, scientific knowledge, and cultural expectations changing at the speed of thought, nursing has become caught between two systems, two cultures, and two paradigms, with one foot firmly planted in the industrial age and one foot in the knowledge age. Nursing's stakeholders are in the same whirlpool of potential disconnect. Instead of honoring both needs and both systems and cultures, nursing has felt pulled, disjointed, and in a functional disarray that has led to cross-discipline competition, jealousy, and elitism, and is becoming known as a profession that "eats its young"—a pretty incongruous personality for a profession that is all about "care"!

What is the difference between a knowledge worker and an industry worker? Both require education and skills, and both must act from a set of competencies. The difference is not between "professional," "paraprofessional," and "vocational," although these terms have been used to describe the differences between advanced practice (AP), registered, and practical nurses. Viewing the professional entities that all describe "nursing" by trying to impose vocational versus professional labels has been one of the central factors contributing to the misunderstanding and tensions among levels of professional nursing.

Let's take a look at the definition of *professional* from the *Oxford Desk Dictionary* (2005): "of, belonging to, or connected to a profession . . . skillful . . . worthy of professional conduct . . . engaged in a specified activity as one's main paid occupation." A *profession* is defined by Oxford as "work requiring specialized advanced training." These definitions encompass every level of nursing, from LPN to AP. The American Nurses Association (ANA) has created a definition of professional nursing as "the promotion, protection and optimization of health and abilities, prevention of illness and injury, alleviation of suffering through the diagnosis and treatment of human response, and advocacy in the care of individuals, families, communities, and populations" (2005).

We would like to propose that the best way to identify the differences in the levels of nursing is to look at the profession's need for nurses who are skilled at the "industry" (skill-based/muscle-reflexor) level and nurses who are skilled at the "knowledge worker" level. One works in direct skill-based care that requires advanced training and education. At the other end of the nursing professional continuum are the nurses whose professional pursuits are based primarily in intellectual endeavor and require even more advanced training and education. All nurses, LPN to AP, are required to demonstrate professional development; continual, lifelong learning is fundamental to the nursing habitat, whether a nurse practices primarily as an industry worker or as a knowledge worker. All nurses provide care based on the diagnosis of the human response.

Perhaps a more appropriate nomenclature is to respect that all nurses are, at every level, professionals; the difference does not reside in "professional" versus "vocational" (defined by Oxford as a trade, or skilled craft). Nursing is nursing at every level; an AP nurse inserts an indwelling catheter the same way, with the same underlying skill and knowledge base, that an LPN does. Principles of medication administration do not change across nursing levels; therapeutic communication is therapeutic communication. What is different is the continuum, from primarily working as a muscle-reflexor (industry worker) to working primarily as a nurse involved in intellectual endeavors (knowledge worker). Each level is cardinal to the extensive and complex profession defined as nursing.

Along that continuum are many ways to nurse: The challenges of ongoing learning and responsiveness are universal, regardless of whether a nurse is an industry worker or a knowledge worker. The drivers of health care will continue to require industry workers—in 2006, there were more than 1500 state-approved training programs in practical nursing, with 26% (194,740) of all LPNs working in hospitals (BLS, 2008b). At the same time, healthcare drivers will call for a greater percentage of knowledge workers. This paradigm shift is evident in how business is being conducted in every sector. The advent of tele-health is a prime example of how nursing must launch a practice environment specialty from a knowledge base.

Today's reality is that nursing is comprised of two systems, two cultures, and two paradigms, with one foot firmly planted in the industrial age and one foot in the knowledge age. That is a good thing; we need both. What nursing needs now is to embrace a new shift and a new set of drivers that will command even greater knowledge, vigor, and initiatives while not excluding or demeaning the value of, and need for, the industry worker. Strategic planning will help to identify these key functions and their unique practice domains, facilitate the process of embracing the industry worker and the knowledge worker, and clarify the mission, goals, and objectives of nursing, today and tomorrow.

THE NATIONAL NURSE, PAY FOR PERFORMANCE, AND MAGNET STATUS

Teri Mills, a nurse educator at Portland Community College in Portland, Oregon, wrote an article in *The New York Times* in May 2005 proposing that the nation have a National Nurse and not just a Surgeon General. The article has caused quite a stir and was instrumental in the House of Representatives' introduction of H.R. 4903 on March 8, 2006. The purpose of a National Nurse will be to:

- Establish symbolic national leadership by elevating and strengthening the Chief Nurse Officer of the USPHS [United States Public Health Service] to make this position visible to the nursing profession and the public.
- Complement the work of the U.S. Surgeon General.
- Promote involvement in the Medical Reserve Corps to improve the health and safety of the community.
- Incorporate proven evidence-based public health education when promoting prevention. (Mills, 2007)

The bill was refereed to the Subcommittee on Health on March 17, 2006, where it remains. A single nurse educator at the community college level has made a significant change in the way we think about a prestigious national office. Imagine what effective strategic planning and implementation from other nurse educators could do for such a cause; the thought of such a powerful and positive force staggers the mind!

Pay for Performance

Have you been evaluated based on competencies? Did you feel that the competencies were truly measurable, definitive, and realistic? Did you have a hand in developing the competency criteria; if not, who did? Have you evaluated anyone else based on a competency model? Skill-based competencies are fairly easy to measure; either the person being evaluated can effectively and efficiently operate the new infusion pump, or he or she can't. Have you been evaluated on a subjective competency, such as "works effectively with patients from diverse backgrounds" or "establishes and maintains rapport"? How does it go when you have to evaluate someone using a subjective parameter? These are important questions to answer. We may be headed toward being paid based on competence; it is called "pay for performance."

The competency model came from work done by a Harvard psychologist, David McClelland, in the 1960s. His hope was to identify an algorithm that could easily recognize the difference between "top performers" and those whose work fell below standards. This body of knowledge has been slow to adapt, but competency-based evaluation began gaining momentum in the 1990s and is continually gathering force. Some arenas of business have already adapted some form of pay scale based on competence.

There are numerous competency models for nursing: Health Leadership, Nursing Leadership, the Diversity Competency Model, the Tennessee Competency Model, the American Nephrology Nurses Association competency model, the Arizona Board of Nursing Competency Model, to name a few. In addition, the ANA has set nine standards of practice that determine general competencies. Given the many ways to practice the profession of nursing, added to the many drivers of care, it is easy to understand the existence and evolution of diverse "competencies."

In the May 2008 issue of *American Nurse Today* (the journal of the ANA), Rebecca Patton, president of the ANA, talked about the value of consumer reports. She compared purchasing health care to the purchase of a new car: She would not do either without consulting safety records and ratings. Ms. Patton cited the goal of CMS as a key driver of quality initiatives, saying, "transform Medicare from a passive payer of claims to an active purchaser of care" (ANA, 2008).

As the largest payer of care for those who are Medicare eligible, CMS sets the trend for healthcare reimbursement. Pay-for-performance (P4P) is one of CMS's initiatives to encourage quality improvement (CMS, 2005). CMS is developing and implementing several sets of P4P models that seek to support quality improvement. In 2007, CMS, as a part of the Deficit Reduction Act of 2005, established several "never events," or serious preventable events that it will no longer reimburse for (Table 2-1).

Should nursing be evaluated solely with a competency set? The jury is still out, but it is looking like we are headed for some type of competency-based model for hiring and promotion criteria and possibly for pay computations. Accrediting bodies are already employing competency-based evaluation models. Competency assessment is a Joint Commission requirement.

Strategic planning requires resource management (ongoing evaluation of resource utilization); the most expensive and difficult to manage is the human resource (recall that nursing is in crisis). Skill and knowledge levels and abilities can only be measured against standards. To create a universally understood set of measurement criteria, those standards are translated into competency sets.

Theoretically, every facility could create a unique set of competencies. We think that it is a very bad idea for nonnurses to dictate nursing. For example, administration should not decide how nursing is "measured"; nursing should measure nursing. Sound strategic planning from within nursing would place the ownership of competency models where they belong: with nursing.

Table 2-1   The CMS Deficit Reduction Act of 2005—Preventable Events

- Object left in surgery.
- Serious Preventable Event—air embolism.
- Serious Preventable Event—blood incompatibility.
- Catheter-associated urinary tract infections.
- Pressure ulcers (decubitus ulcers).
- Vascular catheter-associated infection.
- Surgical site infection—mediastinitis after coronary artery bypass graft surgery.
- Hospital-acquired injuries—fractures, dislocations, intracranial injury, crushing injury, burns, and other causes.

Source: UAB Health System, 2007.
Have you known of any of these occurrences? Please see http://www.cms.hhs.gov/apps/media/press/release.asp?counter=1343 to learn more about the P4P quality initiatives from CMS that continue to impact nursing's habitat.

In 1998, the Pew Health Professions Commission (housed at the University of San Francisco) set 21 competencies for healthcare workers in the 21st century (Table 2-2).

The full report, *Recreating Health Professional Practice for a New Century*, can be found at http://www.futurehealth.ucsf.edu/pdf_files/recreate.pdf. These are generic competencies that are transferable across healthcare disciplines but embedded in competency models designed for nursing.

The ANA has developed the *Continuing Professional Nursing Competence Process* (Whittaker, Smolneski, & Carson, 2000). In the *Online Journal of Issues in Nursing*, Carrie Lenburg (1999) wrote, "In recent years, a critical mass of society's leaders, policy makers, gatekeepers, and stakeholders in

Table 2-2   Pew Health Professionals Commission Competencies for Healthcare Workers

1. Embrace a personal ethic of social responsibility and service.
2. Exhibit ethical behavior in all professional activities.
3. Provide evidence-based, clinically competent care.
4. Incorporate the multiple determinants of health in clinical care.
5. Apply knowledge of the new sciences.
6. Demonstrate critical thinking, reflection, and problem-solving skills.
7. Understand the role of primary care.
8. Rigorously practice preventive health care.
9. Integrate population-based care and services into practice.
10. Improve access to health care for those with unmet health needs.
11. Practice relationship-centered care with individuals and families.
12. Provide culturally sensitive care to a diverse society.
13. Partner with communities in healthcare decisions.
14. Use communication and information technology effectively and appropriately.
15. Work in interdisciplinary teams.
16. Ensure care that balances individual, professional, system, and societal needs.
17. Practice leadership.
18. Take responsibility for quality of care and health outcomes at all levels.
19. Contribute to continuous improvement of the healthcare system.
20. Advocate for public policy that promotes and protects the health of the public.
21. Continue to learn and help others learn.

Source: http://www.futurehealth.ucsf.edu/pewcomm/competen.html

health care and other disciplines has become increasingly concerned and ready to engage in serious debate about competency issues, in the interest of the public good and global competition." Competency models are here to stay; nurses must be actively involved in their evolution and maturation as drivers of practice.

At the Call to the Nursing Profession summit in 2001, leaders from more than 60 national nursing organizations created an in-depth strategic plan, *Nursing's Agenda for the Future* (Nursing World, 2002). They created a vision for nursing in 2010. The document is organized around 10 domains: leadership and planning, economic value, delivery systems/delivery models, work environment, legislation/regulation/policy, public relations/communication, professional/nursing culture, education, recruitment/retention, and cultural diversity. This plan was circulated to many nursing organizations. Do you know what it says, and do you know where nursing "is" in relation to the vision for 2010?

> Please see http://www.nursingworld.org/MainMenuCategories/Healthcare andPolicyIssues/Reports/AgendafortheFuture.aspx to read the strategic planning report.

There is dialogue at healthcare boardroom tables around the country that a partial solution to the chasms in care and the nursing crisis could be addressed by pay for performance (i.e., competency-based evaluation). The extent of such an undertaking is very complex, and nursing must be *the* leader in this dialogue. Having clear and competent skills and knowledge of the strategic planning process is foundational to entering into this discussion and decision-making process. Nursing knows that quality is the highest standard of care; nursing hasn't always known how to overcome the barriers to that quality.

> Remember, empowerment is not solely about achieving competence within scope of practice; empowerment flows from the ability to effect positive change based on that scope of competence—nursing stays on the periphery if it is not fully engaged in the boardrooms.

Magnet Status

Are you attracted, like a magnet, to your hospital? Are the work environment, quality indicators, and nursing leadership so compellingly wonderful that this is the best place to work ever? Magnet Status involves a set of criteria that establishes a hospital as a "best place for nurses to work." Fourteen "forces of magnetism" were identified through a task force study conducted by the American Academy of Nursing (AAN) in 1983. These forces set apart those hospitals designated as Magnet by their ability to attract and retain "professional" nurses.

The next step in the process of developing a Magnet credential came when the American Nurses Credentialing Center (ANCC) was established in 1990 through the ANA. The landmark project of the ANCC was to develop the Magnet Hospital Recognition Program for Excellence in Nursing, based on the 1983 work of the AAN. In 1997, the name of the program changed to Magnet Nursing Services Recognition Program. The program is based on the ANA's Scope and Standards of Practice for Nursing Administrators. A revised draft (second edition) of these standards was released in 2007. The market brand for this initiative was deemed Magnet Status®.

So, how does this impact your practice, the practice of your students, peers, and subordinates, and the profession as a whole? What does this initiative mean for the future of nursing? An interesting distinction made in the definition is that Magnet hospitals attract "professional" nurses; is there any other kind? Does that mean that nonprofessional nurses are working somewhere else? The tenets and concepts of magnetism are brilliant, vital, and exciting, but can every place a nurse works really fit into the ANCC's credentialing criteria? If a healthcare facility or system does not meet Magnet Status, does that mean that those nurses are "less than" nurses who work within a Magnet system? For that matter, should any nurse work in anything less than a facility or system that seeks excellence for all involved?

The Magnet credentialing process leaves out most long-term care nurses, virtually all clinic nurses, many public health and community nurses, school nurses, small hospital nurses, rural and frontier nurses, and even parish nurses; the fact is, the industry realities and economics simply do not exist to support Magnet Status in any but the wealthiest medical centers.

Now, imagine a strategic plan that conceptualizes a magnetism model for those areas of health care that are facing the greatest challenges in attracting and retaining nurses. Nowhere are the plight of dissatisfaction, high turnover, and quality chasms more greatly felt than with nurses who choose to work in long-term care/nursing centers, yet the demographic shifts and trends render the profession of gerontology nursing essential, challenging on every horizon, and a cavity of "crisis." Today, magnetism is for the already-privileged healthcare entities; a sound strategic plan could broaden the vision to include all nurses in all practice settings.

Please visit http://www.nursecredentialing.org to learn more about Magnet Status.

THE NEW GLOBAL FRONTIER—IS NURSING PART OF THE DISCOVERY, OR SAFE AT HOME ALL CUDDLED IN WHITE?

Just a little over 30 years ago, nurses wore white—usually a white dress and white stockings, and caps with distinguishing stripes—and proudly displayed their school pin. Some nurses still wore the navy blue capes with a red satin lining. The hat had to be starched and the dress below the knee, with long sleeves and a high collar. Shoes were inspected for daily polish, and nails were inspected for length (short) and hygiene. Graduation ceremonies included the Nightingale Pledge, candle lighting, and a passing of the flame (symbolizing the Lady of the Lamp) from one generation of nurses to another. The pomp and circumstance was magnificent—an honor and a privilege.

But somewhere in the last three decades, nursing has lost some of its identifying rituals, and its culture has become somewhat fuzzy. Nursing was a younger profession then, and it is only right that as the profession grows, matures, and changes, growing pains are felt.

And it is not surprising that nurses are a little weary of responding to all the trendy and hip directions that have been set by peers, regulatory and advisory bodies, and the tides of time itself. New learning, evidence-based care, and best practices are wonderful, but the many new theories models, management styles, and administrators and their newfangled techniques have been exhausting; they aren't all that great, and they've been imposed on nursing like a juggling act.

What we are witnessing is nursing's loss of identity in a cacophony of global drivers. The loss of identity has led to a veering off the path that encapsulated the values and vision of the "Ladies of the Lamp" and what it means to be a nurse. Nursing has gotten sidetracked. In her book, *Nursing Against the Odds: How Health Care Cost Cutting, Media Stereotypes, and Medical Hubris Undermine Nurses and Patient Care* (2005), Suzanne Gordon talked about the "denursification" of the developed world.

Denursification is clear imagery for a serious crisis. How do we attend to the challenges of change, growth, and maturity—and drivers such as healthcare financing—while maintaining the best of what it means to be a nurse? Yes, we do have an idea; strategic planning starts with clear values and seeks to implement a clear vision. Denursification is a result of fuzzy thinking, unclear values, and even fuzzier vision.

Denursification exists universally, but that does not mean that nursing has completely lost its way. Yes, there are a plethora of drivers, yes, nursing is in crisis, and yes, there are a boatload of challenges facing nursing. We have felt denursified and pulled off center from our core values and vision for nursing; it isn't too hard to get led astray when patient loads, staff shortages, excessively lean budgets, and complex care paradigms are the order of the day.

The business end of the stick may have been part of nursing's derailment, but that very stick can get nursing back on track. We may not go back to starched white anythings, but we may need to recapture and refine nursing's identity and create meaningful new cultural rituals for the 21st century— smart, responsive, and organizationally sound rituals, just like those of any business organization.

The New Global Frontier

If nursing has lost some of its identity, how can it be clear about its role in a global healthcare arena? The *new global frontier* is a term coined by business to define a complex global economy and all the resources (not the least of which is the human resource) that constitute management of all affairs. The global frontier impacts health care every day. Exactly where does nursing fit strategically in a global economy? Is nursing a minor player, a major participant, a decision-maker, a change agent, a leader, a manager, a follower, or a chief executive officer (CEO) at the helm of care?

> We would like you to take a moment here to answer these very important questions:
>
> - What do you think nursing's role should be in the global frontier of the 21st century?
> - Have you considered your purpose as a nurse?
> - How do you see yourself? As a minor player, major participant, decision-maker, change agent, leader, manager, follower, or CEO? Other?

These questions are imperative to answer. All directions must begin with a clear view of purpose. Nursing's identity has gotten a little fuzzy; we are not clad-in-white industry workers, but we are not solely knowledge workers. Levels of nursing have created parameter territory wars; we need all nurses, but we need to be clear about why each is here. If nursing is to be a cardinal constituent of care, every nurse must have a crystal clear conviction of the meaning and intent of care.

As an example, here is Michele's purpose statement: "To inspire and empower nurses and nursing to actualize their highest vision of care in order to heal the world and create peace and possibility for the world's children."

What is your purpose statement? How would you tell someone about the purpose of nursing? How would you define nursing? How do you define care?

Florence Nightingale, in her book *Notes on Nursing: What It Is and What It Is Not*, speaks of care in relation to sanitation and observation. Her purpose was to "give hints for thought to women who have personal charge of the health of others" (Nightingale, 1860/1960, p. xi). In the early 1900s, Mary Breckenridge dedicated her life to helping women and children. She created the Frontier Nursing Service (FNS) and, in 1939, the FNS School of Midwifery and Family Nursing. Her purpose was to improve the health and well-being of women and children where maternal and child deaths were the highest in the country. Lillian Wald, a nurse in the early 1900s, defined nursing as "love in action, and there is no finer manifestation of it than the care of the poor and disabled in their own homes" (Wald, n.d.). The first model for home health care came from work done by Ms. Wald. These are just three examples of nurses who had clear vision and purpose. These three courageous women—courageous nurses—had a clear purpose, a good plan, and terrific implementation skills. They may not have called their process "strategic planning," but that is exactly how they got from where they were to where they wanted to be.

The challenges of this new global frontier are daunting. We think white is a dumb color choice for a potentially messy career. Starch is really uncomfortable. Denursification has happened and is happening. Nursing has had some amazing leaders. Sadly, many of our leaders today are embroiled in theories, politics, and power—kind of cuddled in white and safe at home. Who are our Mary Breckinridges and Lillian Walds, and how do we help them face and meet the challenges of this new global frontier without getting tangled in support stockings and IV tubing? Purpose—clear purpose based on clear values. Florence, Mary, and Lillian had values and purpose in abundance; they certainly were not all cuddled in white and safe at home.

A NEW HEALTH SYSTEM FOR THE 21ST CENTURY

The Institute of Medicine (IOM) undertook a campaign to understand and communicate the disparities in health care; from this work, several documents expounding on the chasms in care have been produced and continue to be researched and written. In one account, *To Err is Human: Building a Safer*

Health System, the IOM reported that at least 98,000 hospitalized Americans die annually as a result of errors in their care (IOM, 2000). In *Keeping Patients Safe: Transforming the Work Environment of Nurses* (IOM, 2004), the IOM goes on to say that the 98,000 deaths represent only those that occur in hospitals; no data are available on deaths that occur in nursing homes, at home (home health), in clinics, in stand-alone surgery centers, in public health facilities, in family planning clinics, and so on. AIDS, motor vehicle fatalities, and breast cancer do not kill as many people as errors in care do. Now there is a sobering consideration: Nurses who are charged with care are part of phenomenal harm. Another alarming conclusion is that the data do not include patients who do not die as a result of error but who were left with a serious injury or a chronic condition. The IOM has established eight select indicators that point to chasms in care (Table 2-3).

The IOM defines quality as "the degree to which health services for individuals and populations increases the likelihood of desired outcomes and are consistent with current professional knowledge" (IOM, 2008). To operationally quantify this definition, the IOM has set 6 aims for improvement and 10 rules (principles) for redesign of healthcare systems (Table 2-4).

Table 2-3   The Institute of Medicine's Indicators That Point to Chasms in Care

1. Between 44,000 and 98,000 Americans die from medical errors annually.
2. Only 55% of patients in a recent random sample of adults received recommended care, with little difference found between care recommended for prevention, care recommended to address acute episodes, or care recommended to treat chronic conditions.
3. Medication-related errors for hospitalized patients cost roughly $2 billion annually.
4. A total of 41 million uninsured Americans exhibit consistently worse clinical outcomes than the insured and are at increased risk for dying prematurely.
5. The lag between the discovery of more effective forms of treatment and their incorporation into routine patient care averages 17 years.
6. A total of 18,000 Americans die each year from heart attacks because they did not receive preventive medications, although they were eligible for them.
7. Medical errors kill more people per year than breast cancer, AIDS, or motor vehicle accidents.
8. More than 50% of patients with diabetes, hypertension, tobacco addiction, hyperlipidemia, congestive heart failure, asthma, depression, and chronic atrial fibrillation are currently managed inadequately.

Source: IOM, 2008.

Table 2-4   The Institute of Medicine's 6 Improvement Initiatives and 10 Rules to Achieve the Initiatives

Improvement initiatives
1. Safe
2. Effective
3. Patient-centered
4. Timely
5. Efficient
6. Equitable

Rules to achieve the initiatives
1. Care is based on continuous healing relationships.
2. Care is customized based on patient needs and values.
3. Patient is the source of control.
4. Knowledge is shared and information flows freely.
5. Decision-making is evidence-based.
6. Safety is a system property.
7. Transparency is necessary.
8. Needs are anticipated.
9. Waste is continuously decreased.
10. Cooperation among clinicians is a priority.

Source: IOM, 2001.

Since the release of the chasm reports beginning in 1999, several other entities have begun earnest work on creating an improved healthcare system. There are three levels within the healthcare system that have their own unique focus for quality improvement, based on the reports from the IOM: the environmental level, the healthcare organization level, and the level at which clinicians and patients interconnect—where care meets the patient. These levels include healthcare organizations, employers and consumers, research foundations, government agencies, and quality improvement organizations.

Have you wondered why every meeting has something to do with "quality"—total quality management (TQM), continuous quality management (CQM), or quality improvement (QI)? It is because the findings from the IOM, as well as other entities, have been driving healthcare financing for almost a decade: Where money flows, so flow priorities. Errors cost consumers over $2 billion per year (IOM, 2004). With nurses providing 60–90% of all care delivered (BLS, 2008b), the onus for error correction and prevention falls heavily on the domain of nursing.

Nursing didn't have to be told that there were gaps in care; we already knew. Well before the IOM reports came out, nursing was pleading for safe staffing levels and to be seen as an asset, not an expendable commodity. In 1994, the ANA instituted the Safety & Quality Initiative to assess the relationship between patient care and patient outcomes.

From this work came the *Nursing Care Report Card for Acute Care* in 1995 (you may order a copy of the report from http://www.nursebooks.org). This report identified 21 measures of care linked to quality and availability of "qualified" (*qualified* is not defined) nursing staff. Three key areas of quality indicators were described (Table 2-5).

It is pretty easy to see that today's nurses have a tremendous amount of work to synthesize and competently implement solutions to these challenges in this 21st-century healthcare environment! We wish Florence, Mary, and Lillian served on the IOM; they would be clear about nursing's role, and they

---

Table 2-5   The American Nurses Association's 21 Measures of Care

1. Patient-focused outcome indicators (six subcategories)
     Mortality rates
     Length of stay
     Adverse events
     Complications
     Patient and family satisfaction
     Patient adherence to discharge plan
2. Process of care indicators (eight subcategories)
     Nurse satisfaction
     Assessment and implementation of patient care
     Pain management
     Maintenance of skin integrity
     Patient education
     Discharge planning
     Assurance of patient safety
     Responsiveness to unplanned patient care needs
3. Structure of care indicators—nurse staffing patterns (seven subcategories)
     Ratio of total nursing staff to patients
     Ratio of RNs to total nursing staff
     RN staff qualifications
     Total nursing care hours provided per patient
     Staff continuity
     RN overtime
     Nursing staff injury rate

How are you and your organization doing with keeping track of these nursing-sensitive indicators? How do you think schools of nursing are doing at imparting and measuring these?

The ANA quality measures were based on what was coined "nursing-sensitive quality measures" (ANA, 1994). These measures evolved into the quality indicators that the National Database of Nursing Quality Indicators (NDNQI) now comprises. The data—compliance and progress toward achieving and maintaining these benchmarks—are reported to the National Quality Forum (NQF). You can learn more about these nursing-sensitive indicators by visiting http://www.nursing quality.org or http://www.qualityforum.org/nursing.

would have a clear strategy! Alas, they are not. So instead of wishing, depending on, and waiting for a few bright stars to close the chasms, wouldn't it be better to include all of nursing in this change and evolution process? Nurses cannot be expected to jump on the change bandwagon and work effectively and efficiently toward the many calls to excellence without process skills. OK, here it is again: We have much work to accomplish. All nurses need to understand change processes, and fundamental to change processes is the understanding of sound strategic planning tools.

INTERNATIONAL NURSING: A 43 MILLION SHORTFALL

We just took a brief, if not somewhat sobering, look at healthcare chasms in the United States, but it pales in comparison to what the conundrums, chasms, disparities, challenges, et al., look like across the globe. Knowing that we don't want to stay all "safe at home all cuddled in white" (we can't, even if we did want to; the world is connected by the speed of the Internet and just one jet flight, not to mention the commodity and financial connections and interdependence), how on earth are we supposed to respond to our nation's healthcare dilemmas and still be—at the minimum ethically—responsive to healthcare troubles beyond our borders? You guessed it: We need a plan!

The Americas have 37% of all health workers, but we only have 10% of the global burden of disease (GBD) (World Health Organization [WHO], 2006). In the United States we have 1000 nurses for every 100,000 population, whereas Sub-Sahara Africa has 10 nurses per 100,000 population (ICN, 2004). Fifty-seven countries, mostly in Africa and Asia, have critical health worker shortages. The world's 6000 schools of nursing simply do not produce enough nurses; more important, they do not produce enough nurses who will be vested in areas of extreme shortages. Our education and training centers either do not partner with these shortage areas, or they do not educate and train a workforce that is competent, in all domains, to live and work in resource-challenged settings. The

WHO (2006) describes this disconnect as a need to "get workers with the right skills to the right place at the right time and improve social compatibility between workers and clients."

Please visit http://www.who.int/healthinfo/global_burden_disease/2004 _report_update/en/index.html to learn more about the strategic plan set out by the WHO to address the GBD and the health workforce.

We have all heard of the atrocious and astounding healthcare data—the AIDS epidemic and its orphans in Africa and Asia; Ebola and hemorrhagic diseases; influenza, pandemic influenza, and other emerging disease threats; starvation and malnutrition; unsafe drinking water; open sewage; death from vaccine-preventable diseases; global warming and its ramifications; the rise in antibiotic-resistant microbes such as tenacious strains of TB; abject poverty; children being used as agents of war; women being intentionally infected with AIDS and used as "weapons" of war; food-borne outbreaks; and biologic and chemical threats. What "data" alarm or frighten you? What do you think that nursing in the United States, or any developed country, has done, can do, or should be doing about healthcare chasms that reach beyond our borders?

World Health Organization

The World Health Organization was created on April 7, 1948, with the signing of its constitution under the United Nations (UN) (WHO, 2008). The WHO is charged with the directing and coordinating authority for health within the United Nations system. It is responsible for providing leadership on global health matters, shaping the health research agenda, setting norms and standards, articulating evidence-based policy options, providing technical support to countries, and monitoring and assessing health trends. In the 21st century, health is a shared responsibility, involving equitable access to essential care and collective defense against transnational threats (WHO, 2008).

Our Centers for Disease Control and Prevention (CDC) partners with the WHO and its many suborganizations (such as the United Nations Children's Fund [UNICEF]). As a member of the UN, our country has a legal declaration of global interrelatedness and obligation. That means "us."

International Council of Nurses

As a member of the ANA, you are also a member of the International Council of Nurses (ICN). Do you know what they are up to? What is the strategic plan for the ICN? What is your part in its implementation? Under the ICN is the International Council for Nursing Practice (ICNP). See Table 2-6 for the ICNP's strategic goals.

The ICN (2008) defines nursing as

> encompass[ing] autonomous and collaborative care of individuals of all ages, families, groups and communities, sick or well and in all settings. Nursing includes the promotion of health, prevention of illness, and the care of ill, disabled and dying people. Advocacy, promotion of a safe environment, research, participation in shaping health policy and in patient and health systems management, and education are also key nursing roles.

How are you doing with the fulfillment of that definition? How do you think nursing universally is doing with the fulfillment of that definition?

Do you know that the international symbol for nursing is a white heart that represents the bringing together of all colors—white as a worldwide association with nurses, hygiene, caring, and comfort, and the heart as a symbol of humanity and the role of nursing in quality care? The authors have been in nursing and nursing education for 49 years collectively, but we didn't know about the white heart until recently. Shouldn't all nurses know about our professional symbol? How do we disseminate that "branding" that articulates our vision and purpose?

Historically, isolationism never worked too well. The "new" way to look at work design is called meta-leadership. Simply stated, we aren't supposed to work in "silos," in isolation from other disciplines and other nurses, doing our own thing. We all need each other; we need nurses in Mozambique, we need corn from South America, we need technology and parts from China, and we need to collaborate *and* lead. The IOM, the WHO, the ANA, the ICN, and many

---

Table 2-6 The International Council of Nurses' Strategic Goals

- Serve as a major force to articulate nursing's contribution to health and health care globally.
- Promote harmonization with other widely used classifications and the work of standardization groups in health and nursing.

Source: ICN, 2008.

other lead agencies are changing the face of the healthcare habitat: Nurses need and have a professional obligation to be a part of that planned change.

Nurses are charged with care and make up the majority of workers in all healthcare settings. Simple logic tells us that some of the onus to address chasms in care—wherever they may be, and on whichever continent they may be—falls squarely on the shoulders of nursing. If our leadership organizations have strategic goals and plans, should we, as members of the culture and profession of nursing, be a part of strategic planning and implementation? Step 1 is that we all learn how to work with and within strategic planning processes and learn organizational skills.

TELECONNECTIONS, TELENURSING, TELE-EVERYTHING

Just in case you are not sure how and why strategic planning fits with nursing and care, let's take a look at rapidly emerging disciplines within nursing: telenursing, which also may be referred to as information technology (IT), informatics, or telehealth.

This is a huge part of the healthcare habitat that is changing at Mach speed. "Worldwide, people living in rural and remote areas struggle to access timely, quality specialty medical care" (Brown, 1995, p. 1). Telehealth is a major piece of the solution set to address access and cost containment challenges, and it is changing the healthcare habitat of nursing.

Although we tend to think of telemedicine (telenursing and telehealth) as relatively new, paralleling the advent of the computer age, it has been around for a very long time. The "father of electrocardiography" (ECG), Willem Einthoven, winner of the Nobel Peace Prize for Medicine in 1924, first experimented with transmitting ECGs over phone lines in 1906 (Giovas, 2008).

War has always had a way of creating from necessity. World War I, from 1914 to 1918, was very much a maritime war; never before had such huge battles been fought from floating decks, but there were not enough physicians to be on every ship. The solution for distant care did not come until the 1920s, when "radio doctors" were located at shore stations. Their job was to help sailors at sea with medical emergencies.

Telepsychiatry has been around since the Nebraska Psychiatric Institute first used closed-circuit TV to assess and monitor patients in 1955. One of the coolest (literally) uses of telemedicine came with the advent of NASA's Landsat satellites in the 1970s, which were used to link emergency medical services in remote Alaskan communities with big city hospitals.

So, if tele-everything has been around so long, why are we just now getting around to implementation? Well, people are slow at adapting to change, and nursing simply did not grab ahold of the concept of "computers in nursing" (also referred to as IT and nursing informatics) because nursing in general "feared and distrusted it; believed [that] it was too complicated for them . . . and . . . would take away their creativity and discourage thinking" (Ronald, 2001).

IT and all its relatives are here to stay. Today, there are more than 25 schools of nursing that offer undergraduate or graduate degrees in nursing informatics (telenursing). The WHO proposes that health workers should be employing IT as a means of greater access to education. The IOM advocates for the use of health information technology. The National League for Nursing (NLN) recently released a position statement, *Preparing the Next Generation of Nurses to Practice in a Technology-Rich Environment: An Informatics Agenda*, stating the importance of competence in "21st century knowledge and skills for practice in a complex, emerging technologically sophisticated, consumer-centric, global environment" (NLN, 2008).

Please see http://www.nln.org/aboutnln/PositionStatements/informatics _052808.pdf to view the complete document. What is your personal position statement on nursing and technology? How do you see technology changing the face of nursing? How should this change be orchestrated (strategically planned)?

ANTICIPATING THE FUTURE OF NURSING

Given the many drivers of care—from our professional organizations to our world leaders in health care, the new global frontier, and technology that reaches ever new levels of sophistication weekly—nursing's habitat will continue to change exponentially. Healthcare futurists abound. But unless the vision and direction of nursing flow from within the ranks of nursing, change will be sporadic and confusing and will breed resentment—just as it has over the past few decades.

We have given you a brief overview of some of the ways the nursing habitat has changed and will continue to change. Perhaps you can think of changes we have overlooked. As we begin to take you through the strategic planning process, you will come to understand the cardinal importance of being "clear why we are here." So instead of us telling you what we think the healthcare environment of the 21st century is going to look like, we want you to begin your own visioning process.

Here are a few questions that we would like you to consider. Get out a big piece of paper and your favorite writing utensil, and let yourself clearly imagine your current vision, and your ideal future vision, of nursing:

(1) What does the work environment for nurses look like to you today? (Consider wages; location; people you work with; hours, days, and shifts; satisfaction; options for advancement or lateral movement; your primary duties and how you spend the majority of your work hours; work design; management styles; leadership; quality of outcomes; and anything else that work "today" feels like.)

(2) What does the work environment for nurses in 5 years look like to you?

(3) What does the work environment for nurses in 20 years look like to you? In 100 years?

(4) Describe your ideal work environment for nurses.

We would love to know your answers to these questions. Please e-mail your responses to michele@nursesfornursesinternational.com or leann@nursesfornursesinternational.com.

Failing to plan is planning to fail (or at least to stay stuck and be left out of the crucial decision-making). Nurses must be leaders in the solution process or remain a victim of other disciplines' designs and mandates. Create the future of nursing that you want to see. Recall M. Gandhi's idiom, "Be the change that you want to see in the world."

REVIEW QUESTIONS

1. What is the proposed purpose of Teri Mills's National Nurse?
2. What is "pay for performance"?
3. Who accredits Magnet hospitals?
4. Explain the term *denursification*.
5. What is the "new global frontier"?
6. What is the purpose of the WHO?
7. Describe how the industry age and knowledge age affect nursing.

REFERENCES

American Nurses Association (ANA). (1994). *The National Database NDNQI® history.* Retrieved April 6, 2009, from http://www.nursingworld.org/MainMenuCategories/ThePracticeofProfessionalNursing/PatientSafetyQuality/Research-Measurement/The-National-Database.aspx

American Nurses Association (ANA). (2005). *Definition of professional nursing.* Silver Spring, MD: Nursebooks.org.

American Nurses Association (ANA). (2008). Scope and standards of practice for nursing administrators. Retrieved April 6, 2009, from http://nursingworld.org/books/pdescr.cfm?CNum=9

Brown, N. (1995). *A brief history of telemedicine.* Retrieved April 6, 2009, from http://tie.telemed.org/articles/article.asp?path=articles&article=tmhistory_nb_tie95.xml

Bureau of Labor Statistics (BLS). (2008a). *Health care.* Retrieved April 6, 2009, from http://www.bls.gov/oco/cg/cgs035.htm

Bureau of Labor Statistics (BLS). (2008b). *Licensed practical and licensed vocational nurses.* Retrieved April 6, 2009, from http://www.bls.gov/oco/ocos102.htm

Bureau of Labor Statistics (BLS). (2008c). *Registered nurses.* Retrieved April 6, 2009, from http://www.bls.gov/oco/ocos083.htm

Centers for Medicaid and Medicare Services (CMS). (2005). *Medicare pay-for-performance (P4P) initiatives.* CMS Office of Public Affairs. Retrieved April 6, 2009, from http://www.cms.hhs.gov/apps/media/press/release.asp?counter=1343

Centers for Medicaid and Medicare Services (CMS). (2008). *National health expenditure data.* Retrieved April 6, 2009, from http://www.cms.hhs.gov/nationalhealthexpenddata

Giovas, P. (2008). *Telemedicine.* Retrieved April 6, 2009, from http://users.forthnet.gr/ath/giovas/telemed

Gordon, S. (2005). *Nursing against the odds: How health care cost cutting, media stereotypes, and medical hubris undermine nursing and patient care.* Ithaca, NY: Cornell University Press.

H.R. 4903: National Nurse Act of 2006, 109th Congress. (2006). *Govtrack.us.* Retrieved April 10, 2009, from http://www.govtrack.us/congress/bill.xpd?bill=h109-4903

Institute of Medicine (IOM). (2000). *To err is human: Building a safer health system.* Washington, DC: National Academies Press.

Institute of Medicine (IOM). (2001). *Crossing the quality chasm: A new health system for the 21st century.* Washington, DC: National Academies Press.

Institute of Medicine (IOM). (2004). *Keeping patients safe: Transforming the work environment for nurses.* Washington, DC: National Academies Press.

Institute of Medicine (IOM). (2008). *The chasm in quality: Select indicators from recent reports.* Washington, DC: National Academies Press.

International Council of Nurses (ICN). (2004). *The global shortage of registered nurses: An overview of issues and actions.* Retrieved April 6, 2009, from http://www.icn.ch/global/shortage.pdf

International Council of Nurses (ICN). (2008). *Strategic goals.* Retrieved April 30, 2009, from http://www.icn.ch/icnp.htm

Lenburg, C. (1999). Redesigning expectations for initial and continuing competence for contemporary nursing practice. *Online Journal of Issues in Nursing, 4*(2). Retrieved November 11, 2008, from http://www.nursingworld.org/MainMenu Categories/ANAMarketplace/ANAPeriodicals/OJIN/TableofContents/Volume41999/ No2Sep1999/RedesigningExpectationsforInitialandContinuingCompetence.aspx

Mills, T. (2007, August 1). *Latest version of policy to create an Office of the National Nurse.* Retrieved April 6, 2009, from http://nationalnurse3.blogspot.com

National League for Nursing (NLN). (2008). *Preparing the next generation of nurses to practice in a technology-rich environment: An informatics agenda.* Retrieved April 6, 2009, from http://www.nln.org/aboutnln/PositionStatements/informatics_052808.pdf

Nightingale, F. (1960). *Notes on nursing: What it is and what it is not.* Toronto, Canada: Dover. (Original work published 1860)

Nursing World. (2002). *Nursing's agenda for the future: A call to the nation.* Retrieved April 6, 2009, from http://www.nursingworld.org/MainMenuCategories/Healthcare andPolicyIssues/Reports/AgendafortheFuture.aspx

Patton, R. (2008, May). From your ANA president. PR, P4R, P4P, VBP. Connecting the dots—with all of the "P's." *American Nurse Today, 3*(5), 1. Retrieved April 6, 2009, from http://www.americannursetoday.com/Media/PublicationsArticle/ana5-Patton-423.pdf

Professional. (2005). In *Oxford Desk Dictionary American Edition.* New York: Oxford University Press.

Ronald, J. (2001). *Evolution of nursing informatics education.* Retrieved April 6, 2009, from http://www2.amia.org/history/presentations/EvolutionOfInformatics.pdf

UAB Health System. (2007). CMS to halt payment for "never events." *UAB Synopsis, 26*(36). Retrieved April 6, 2009, from http://www.uabhealth.org/33800

Wald, L. D. (n.d.). *Profiles in caring: Lillian D. Wald 1867–1940.* Retrieved April 9, 2009, from http://www.nahc.org/NAHC/Val/Columns/SC10-4.html

Whittaker, S., Smolenski, M. C., & Carson, W. (2000, June 30). Assuring continued competence—Policy questions and approaches: How should the profession respond? *Online Journal of Issues in Nursing, 5*(3). Retrieved April 6, 2009, from www.nursingworld .org/MainMenuCategories/ANAMarketplace/ANAPeriodicals/OJIN/TableofContents/ Volume52000/No3Sept00/ArticlePreviousTopic/ContinuedCompetence.aspx

World Health Organization (WHO). (2006). *The World Health Report 2006: Working together for health.* Geneva, Switzerland: Author.

World Health Organization (WHO). (2008). *History of WHO.* Retrieved April 6, 2009, from http://www.who.int/about/history/en/index.html

The Business That We Find Ourselves In

THE BUSINESS THAT WE FIND OURSELVES IN

Who is reading industry and market changes and who isn't? Who calculates a nurse's worth? How do business principles play into nursing practice? How is nursing promoted, branded, and "sold"? What is nursing's "market position" or "strategic position"? (Do we want one?) These are some of the questions answered by this chapter, which takes a broad view of the umbrella of business that so significantly impacts all that nursing does.

Business is _____ (please fill in the blank). We are nurses, what do we know of "business"? We're not trying to be flippant, but we nurses simply do not have any *real* business skills and knowledge; we have *nursing* skills and knowledge. If you are a graduate-level nurse or higher, we are pretty sure that you got drug through a healthcare financing course and perhaps a management course or two, but business degrees from Harvard we do not have. Can a couple of business-related courses truly prepare you, or any nurse, to work in the *business* of health care? Sure they can, if all we want to do is hang on to the periphery of decision-making; our job, after all is care, not cash-flow projections (or is it?).

Right out of the chute here, we are going to send you to an authority source on business: We have started two successful businesses and are in the start-up phase of another, but we are not business experts. So, before we launch into the content of this chapter, please peruse a copy of the *Harvard Business Review* (a monthly journal), or visit its blog at http://discussionleader.com and take a look at what true business leaders are saying about the paradigms of the 21st century (remember—health care, care, is a business).

There are some very smart ideas out there that can positively impact your personal professional world and the larger arena where you practice your profession. We are not suggesting that we all need an MBA from Harvard, but we sure need to know what's up with the world of business forecasters, trendsetters, and the business principles that drive the profession of care. We need to understand the language, the basic concepts, and the rules of the business process.

Many of the workforce ills in nursing flow from the very real disconnect between *business* and *care*: Care (the "business" of nurses) requires that all nurses have some fundamental understanding and basic competencies surrounding business. We respect that business and care can and have collided, but the reality is that we like getting paid, having benefits, and advancing our careers. That makes nurses, who work in the largest U.S. industry, employing 14 million people (BLS, 2008), very much "in business." A traditional definition of *business* is: "an entity that brings together time, effort and capital in order to produce a profit" (Kenny, 2008). Even nonprofits must pay their bills, pay their employees, and keep a roof over their heads. Let's devilify business and learn how to better work with and within the entities that pay our rent and our mortgages.

A BRIEF HISTORY OF WHEN AND HOW CARE MERGED WITH BUSINESS

Nurses have always worked in some form of care and in some form of establishment. A care establishment is that place where nurses ply their trade and practice their profession. Care establishments come in many forms, but for 59% of all RNs (1,475,000) and 26% (194,740) of all LPNs in the United States today, their care establishment is a hospital (BLS, 2008). The next largest employer of nurses is a long-term care (LTC) facility, where 26% (194,740) of LPNs and 5% (125,000) of RNs are practicing their profession (BLS, 2008). Clinics or physicians' offices are a close third, with 289,880 nurses (12% of LPNs and 8% of RNs) (BLS, 2008). Nurses are also employed in community settings (e.g., public health, school nursing, and home health), in clinics, in outpatient centers, at government agencies and social assistance agencies, and in education, and 4% work in employment services (BLS, 2008).

Gradually (over a few centuries or so), care establishments have shifted from a community-based profession to a primarily hospital-based profession. The first care establishments started in Ancient Egyptian times (the pyramids were places of "cure"; mummies have been discovered that show signs of bone healing after brain surgery!). The early Greeks believed in the healer-god Asclepius. Their hospitals were places where folks came to wait for guidance from Asclepius in a dream. Most hospitals historically formed around war; the nurses, especially in medieval times, were men (strong enough to hold the knight down while his leg was being sawed off—no pesky female traits such as fainting, and certainly no proper woman would ever see unclothed anything!). "Poor houses" and homes for the infirm (weak and sickly) were run by religious organizations and relied on volunteers. Our modern-day word *hospital* comes from the Latin word *hospes*, which means "host," because many early hospitals "hosted" the people no one else wanted or could care for. Amazingly, the remains of the oldest hospital in the world are in Sri Lanka and date from the 4th century B.C.

Thinking of this rich and long history of care, added to the amazing diversity of today's healthcare arena, it is hard to specify all the types of care provided and how nursing is practiced. Nurses provide care in a myriad of care modalities, from military trauma to occupational preventive health and safety, to education, to agricultural health and safety (there are actually trauma courses on how to extricate someone from a piece of farm machinery!). Settings where a nurse can work are also hard to specify; nurses can work in a factory, a school, in the armed services, in the community, in a jail, with a church, on Capitol Hill, or in the barrios of West Los Angeles; all are nurses, all require the same Board of Nursing approval, and all are practicing care.

People have been in the care business for a long time! But what has shifted is the structure in which care is provided: Where once altruism and charity were the hosts of care, business is now the host of care. The business model has not been around all that long. In the past 30 or so years, health care has evolved to be driven by reimbursement models; the drivers with the greatest impact were first the creation of Medicare and Medicaid in 1965 and the Balanced Budget Act (BBA) of 1997.

BUSINESS MODELS OF CARE

Let's look at how the business models of today's health care came about. This will help us to better understand the process, the players, and the healthcare arena (business) that has evolved and that as a result of this process will continue to evolve—the business that we find ourselves in.

Medicare and Medicaid came into existence in 1965 as Title XVIII and Title XIX, respectively, of the Social Security Act. The purpose was to extend health coverage to most Americans over 65 years of age and to provide health services to low-income children who did not have parental support and to those children's caretakers/relatives, the elderly, the blind, and people with disabilities. The elderly continue to be the population most likely to live in poverty. By July 1, 1966, more than 19 million people enrolled in Medicare. In 1972, Medicare expanded to include individuals under 65 with long-term disabilities and end-stage renal disease. In this same year, the Supplemental Social Security program was enacted, allowing Medicaid eligibility for the elderly, blind, and disabled. The year 1973 saw the development of health maintenance organizations (HMOs), which sought to provide quality comprehensive benefits based on federal standards; qualifying HMOs then received preferential treatment in the marketplace as models for Medicare and Medicaid reimbursement. The year 1977 saw the creation of the Health Care Financing Administration (HCFA). In 2001, the HCFA became the Centers for Medicare and Medicaid (CMS) to change the agency's 24-year image as a miserly hoarder of federal monies (meant to stave off fraud and abuse)—not a user-friendly image (Stoil, 2001). The year 1983 saw the implementation of diagnostic-related groups (DRGs) to replace cost-based payments. The year 1988 saw some big changes with the Medicare Catastrophic Act, which dramatically expanded what and whom Medicare would cover—only to be repealed in 1989 and replaced with yet another new Medicare fee schedule.

No nurse can forget the implementation of the Health Insurance Portability and Accountability Act (HIPAA) in 1996. With the onslaught of HIPAA came a drudgery of disconnected in-services as everyone sought to understand the implications of this new process of "portability." The next hallmark for CMS came with the BBA in 1997; this was a major overhaul for reimbursement structures. The largest consequence was the requirement for CMS to develop and implement five new prospective payment systems that would define how Medicare paid for inpatient services, rehabilitation hospital services, home health services, hospital outpatient services, and outpatient rehabilitation services (CMS, 2008).

The Clinton Administration's answer to the recession years of the 1980s came with the BBA. In 1997, the BBA changed the healthcare storefront, the marketing plan, the method of revenue forecasting, gap analysis, and reimbursement models for care. This plan was implemented over a 5-year period (1998–2002) and applied to healthcare providers who treated disabled and senior patients (approximately 36% of all acute care patients are 65 years and older; Nagamine, Jaing, & Merrill, 2006). In 1997, Medicare and Medicaid paid for 54% of all hospital stays (Nagamine et al., 2006) and 61% of total nursing home expenditures (Harrington, 2007). The rising (ongoing) cost of caring for elders and the disabled was addressed by an intricate design of justifications for payment and protocol regarding how care would be paid for—reimbursement via a complex new system of formulas that were meant to save Medicare $116 billion and Medicaid $11 billion in that 5-year period (Barakat, 2000).

Did you notice how many home health agencies, rehabilitation units, and outpatient services disappeared from 1998 to 2002? Did you also notice the increase in paperwork and justification for reimbursement? Why does CMS wield so much control over what happens in the healthcare financing arena? Because where CMS—as the gold standard for healthcare reimbursement—goes, third-party payers (insurance companies) follow. Recall that 54% of all hospital claims in 1997 were paid by CMS, and today, 61% of all nursing home expenditures are paid through CMS.

Although the DRG system, first instituted in 1967 with the introduction of Medicare, had been around for a while, it did not come into full force until the HCFA fully adopted the DRG system in 1983. The DRG reimbursement model was created as a research project by Dr. Fetter (2001) and his research team at Yale University; its aim was to curb ever-increasing acute care costs by cutting Medicaid and Medicare payments. It wasn't meant to be a perfect system, just a piece of the solution. Because no other models existed, the DRG system was adopted with all its perfections and imperfections. It is still evolving today.

Some of the codes used to capture reimbursement under the DRG model have come under serious scrutiny. For example, the coding used by physicians (Current Procedural Terminology, or CPT) was referred to as a monopoly in 2002 by Department of Public Health and Human Services Secretary Thompson (Thompson, 2002) and became fodder for many courtroom debates. (Coding systems are important because they direct literally billions of dollars each year from payers and patients to providers, so controlling those codes is a very big deal. CPT is a registered trademark of the American Medical Association.) The debate surrounding the Medicare conversion factors continues because many providers now refuse to take Medicare clients.

The pendulum of reimbursement has been swinging wildly since 1965, and it doesn't look to be slowing down any time soon.

While intricate rules for reimbursement were made for elder care and for the disabled, Title XXI, the Children Health Insurance Program (CHIP), was created with the BBA to improve access to care for children. Children continue to need access to care (for example, in Montana 44% of all children are uninsured) and "for all children under 18, the poverty rate increased from 16.7 percent in 2002 to 17.6 percent in 2003" (U.S. Census Bureau, 2004). In the period from 2002–2003 the number in poverty rose from 12.1 million to 12.9 million. Coincidentally, what is happening to the American demographic? We are a graying country; this demographic trend has been referred to as the "graying of America," and if you are more alarmed by the trend, you may refer to it as the "gray tsunami." On both ends of the healthcare spectrum, health care and the payment models created to fund the system will continue to evolve, morph, and be recreated. Nursing is intimately involved in this process and must intimately be involved in the planning and challenges of healthcare financing.

PUTTING A PRICE TAG ON NURSING'S PRODUCT: CARE

The nurse's product—time, effort, and capital—is straightforward: Nurses provide care. One of the greatest reasons to be a nurse is the opportunity to practice that care in a multitude of ways, across international boarders, across gender, and across ages. Care can be practiced in a classroom, in an operating room, in a home, or at the bedside. Care that combines time, effort, and capital to equal economic gain determines nursing's price tag: The higher the gain, the higher the price tag. Does this sound familiar? It should; this is the basis of the principle of supply and demand. Another term for this principle is the principle of compensation, which states that profit flows when enough people want what you offer (your product = care).

Is one "type" of nurse more valuable than another? We don't think so, but culturally, hospital nurses have come out ahead on the average pay scales (for example, an RN in a hospital makes an average of $3.57 more per hour than his or her LTC counterpart [BLS, 2008], who may be responsible for as many as 40 clients and is probably the director of nursing as well; who is working harder, more skilled, and more specialized?).

The answer really does not have much to do with which nurse in which setting is "better than" the other, even though that is how it has become viewed within the culture of nursing. If able to respond honestly, most nurses would say that an intensive care unit (ICU) nurse is a "better" nurse than an LTC nurse, and that the ICU nurse has more professional clout than most other nurses. The business of health care has imposed a random price tag on the profession of care; that price tag has been taken to heart by the profession, and a false value system has been both imposed and adopted.

It is outside business forces that have determined the "value" of a nurse; the value is not in the way a nurse practices care. This is very important to understand. False values have been assigned to nurses based on the economics of where they work and not necessarily on the value or lack of value (skill and knowledge) of their area of work; the value discussion has become intricately tied to where the money is. It really comes down to, "Is the specialty area a money maker, or isn't it?" Nurses in high-revenue-potential fields (and coincidentally, high liability areas) make more money. More money equals more clout. More clout equals greater perceived value, and so the cycle goes. This isn't a bad thing, unless you consider what it has done to the culture of nursing or unless you are a nurse who works outside of high-revenue areas. Where is the shortage most greatly felt? It is felt most greatly in gerontology and in rural, frontier, and low-income neighborhoods and settings. It is no coincidence that some of our greatest nursing shortage areas are also where income potential is lower and the least stable. And while federal and state grant monies have expanded the area of gerontology research, there has been no corresponding influx of RNs into LTC or assisted living.

This discussion is in no way meant to lessen the remarkable skills, talents, and knowledge that an ICU nurse must have, but think about why ICU nurses get paid more; yes, they must be exceptional at what they do, but the bottom line is that they work in a unit that is very revenue intense. *All* nurses must be exceptional at what they do; that is the market standard. On the flip side of the coin, in 2002, *The New York Times* reported that "9 out of 10 nursing homes lack adequate staffing" (Pear, 2002): "The Bush administration, citing the costs involved, says it has no plans to set minimum staffing levels for nursing homes . . . hoping instead the problem will be resolved through market forces" (Pear, 2002). What market forces? Recall that time + effort + capital = profit = business; LTC simply does not fit that definition.

What nurses do and where is important to this business discussion because nursing, with its amazing kaleidoscope of possibilities for care, has come to define itself on a value scale based on economics. The economic value of a nurse depends on the setting. Another way to look at this is to say that *only* 59% of all RNs work in a hospital; 41% of all RNs work in other settings. Look anywhere; the majority of research, continuing education, standards, guidelines, and organized efforts to communicate with and improve nursing are focused on hospital nursing. Why? Because efforts flow to where the money is. Take a look at any business, and you will see that probable economic benefit comes first. Burger Queen will not come into a community or neighborhood unless there is a sufficient economic demographic to support the sale of X number of hamburgers. Hospitals and clinics do the same thing: They locate in areas where there is a sufficient population that is covered by insurance and/or financially well-off.

HOW NURSES GET PAID

Hospitals, indeed all healthcare entities, come in three main varieties: for-profit, government, and not-for-profit. For-profit has taken the lead as the majority of hospitals nationwide. For-profits have tested many models for profitability, including managed care and HMOs. Teaching and university-affiliated hospitals usually fall under the for-profit model. The Veterans Administration has the largest government hospital and clinic system. "Free" clinics, general hospitals, and community-owned hospitals are often funded by federal, state, or local monies, or all three. Nonprofit healthcare entities are often owned by religious organizations or philanthropic groups, such as the Shriners Hospitals for Children and St. Jude Children's Research Hospital.

Many healthcare facilities have tried to maintain their founding heritage of charity by combining profit and nonprofit models into their mission statement. Nationally, this marriage of charity and profit can even be seen in the credit card industry: "Americans are becoming more charitable" (Steuerle, 2007). It is a model that many healthcare entities employ. With $28.8 billion in unpaid medical bills in 2005 (Wall, 2007), a charitable model may also be financially savvy, given the many deductions and benefits that come with being a 501(c) (the Internal Revenue Service code for 28 types of nonprofit organizations that may claim exemptions from some federal income taxes). Wall reported in 2007 that, contrary to what one would expect, bad debt is not on the rise nationally because hospitals are categorizing more and more unpaid claims as "charity" (Wall, 2007).

The topic of how and if health care gets paid is a huge issue. Nurses are paid because the billing department is able to collect enough money to pay wages. If $28.8 billion was left uncollected in 2005, imagine that number today, with higher insurance premiums, higher deductibles, and fewer insured. You know those bill collection agencies, with their harsh tactics? They are only 10% effective in collecting "bad debt" (Wall, 2007). If people cannot afford health insurance, how likely is it that they will be able to pay today's healthcare costs? In a 2000 article in the *Journal of the American College of Surgeons*, researchers found that the average hospital stay costs $17,734 (Taheri, Butz, & Greenfield, 2000). Healthcare costs have been driven higher and higher by the cost of technology, liability costs, insurance costs, reimbursement models, new diseases and resistant strains, the cost of producing medications, and the continually rising cost of living.

In the short period from 2005 to 2006, the number of uninsured rose by 2.2 million, from 15.3% of the population to 15.8% (47 million; National Coalition on Health Care, 2006). If that number continues to grow at the rate forecasters are predicting, by 2010, 18% of the population will be uninsured, or 55 million Americans. The other bad news with this projection is that many of the uninsured will be children and young adults.

> Let's look at this from the angle of the Burger Queen example given earlier: To pay its employees, cover overhead costs (the cost of equipment, materials, and services necessary to conduct business, such as electricity, rent, phone/Internet, insurance, wages, taxes, and so on), and make money (recall, business is time + effort + capital = profit), Burger Queen needs to sell 100 hamburgers each week at $2 each. If Burger Queen accepts checks, 20% of the checks will not be collectable. Now Burger Queen will need to sell 120 hamburgers to cover the original 20% bad checks, plus 24 more hamburgers (144 now), to cover the new increase created by the 20% bad checks! This is why the world created actuaries— incredible mathematicians who are whizzes at accounting and statistics and capable of predicting the number of hamburgers to be sold based on the overhead. They factor in bad debt, market conditions like mad cow disease, inflation, and economic indicators, and statistical analysis of how the global economy will respond to whether Burger Queen uses pickles! Imagine if we added accepting credit cards to our little Burger Queen formula of 100 hamburgers at $2 each! We'll leave that to an actuary! The obvious solution to bad debt and/or inability to pay from a few is to increase costs for "everybody else"—and that is pretty much what has happened in health care.

This creates another set of time + effort + capital = profit problems because insurance companies and CMS are not naïve about what health care costs or should cost. Prior to 1983, most health care was billed pretty much as cost (fee) for service: A healthcare entity billed CMS $10 for a Band Aid, and CMS paid $10. Today, elaborate fee schedules define ceilings on how much that band-aid can cost. Effectively, supply is limited while demand is not, and healthcare providers are caught in the gap.

In our Burger Queen analogy, we needed to sell 100 hamburgers at $2 each to be profitable and pay overhead. Now we have bad debt and have to increase sales to 144 hamburgers (we asked our workers to produce more in the same amount of time, hence the rise in the world of "efficiency experts"). Other costs, like plain old inflation, fuel costs for bun delivery, and insurance costs (our competitor, Burger Prince, was sued by a patron for a freezer burn from an ice cream cone, so our liability insurance doubled) now mean that Burger Queen must sell 175 hamburgers without increasing overhead. (Yes, bring back the efficiency experts—we need to get more hamburgers out of those same employees!)

Our customers, Mr. & Mrs. CMS, have a limited budget and have estimated that they will pay $2 for a hamburger, so we cannot raise the price of our hamburger; we simply must make more hamburgers with the same number of employees and maintain the same overhead in order to survive in today's economy. Here is where the foundational economic theory of supply and demand comes in. *Supply* is the amount of product (hamburgers) that Burger Queen is willing and able to sell at a specified price, and *demand* is the number of hamburgers that Mr. & Mrs. CMS are willing and able to buy at $2 each.

Understanding insurance, payment structures, and how nurses get paid is vital to our understanding of the business end of the stick: Wage structures are influenced by available revenue streams and are less influenced by the amount of work, skill, or knowledge. If LTC suddenly became demanded (that market force President Bush referred to), well reimbursed, and well marketed, the wages for nurses working in LTC would rise. The true indicator of increasing wage-to-work ratios is the principle of compensation—the product must *satisfy a need or desire*, the *product offered must be exceptional*, and those offering that product must be really good at *marketing that product*.

Now this is where it can get a little tricky. Who is the *customer* of care who needs care, who sets the standard for "exceptional," and who is the ideal customer to be courted through marketing? Is it CMS (and other payers), or is it the patient? Let's get back to our Burger Queen crew. Now Mr. & Mrs. CMS bring in their children for a hamburger. Whose desire or need must be satisfied in order to sell hamburgers? CMS junior may exert a great deal of influence over where he gets his hamburger, so junior is your customer; however, Mom & Dad CMS may have the final say, so they are your customer too. Health care really does have two customers: the patient, and those who pay the patient's bill. You already know this. Think of all of the regulatory paperwork that must be completed. You're not doing that because the patient will be healthier; you are doing it because you have two clients: the one you give care to, and the ones who pay for that care (the one who ultimately pays the majority of your wages).

Perhaps if more nurses understood this dynamic, there would be less resistance to the perceived burden of paperwork. That paperwork certainly has changed over the past several years. This has been driven in large part by the BBA of 1997 and the cascade of regulations that sought to implement the national plan for tightening our national proverbial healthcare overspending belt.

To review, health care is the largest U.S. industry, employing 14 million people in 2006, with a projection of 3 million more jobs through 2016; it is also the fastest growing U.S. industry (BLS, 2008). In 2001, total healthcare spending reached $1.4 trillion (Levit et al., 2003), and that figure continues to grow. Health care is a gargantuan industry, with many people and entities trying to carve out a piece of healthcare's huge revenue streams. Some seek to "do good" (nonprofit), some seek to serve (government), some seek to profit (forprofit), and some seek a combination of charity, service, and profit. It is a complicated business that we work in, and it will continue to add layers of complexity as the many stakeholders exert influence over the system that is nursing's professional home. If nurses want substantive say in what their product is worth and how they will be paid, they must understand who pays for what and why, and be actively and intelligently involved in the ongoing systems process. You guessed it—nurses must be involved in planning!

Congratulations—you made it through the assault of business and care. Time for a little reprieve to attend to our affective sides; we are, after all, *nurses*. Thomas Lynch (1987) wrote this beautiful passage about the "gifts" of women, but we think that it applies nicely to nurses: "Most days I recite a litany of gratitudes for the pleasures of [women's {nurse's?}] company, the beauty and beatitudes of their intellections. Mine and I have been saved and comforted, challenged and loved and mightily improved by the knowledge of them" (with permission of the author).

RECOMMENDED READING

To further your study of business and business principles, we have included here some recommended reading:

1. Drucker, P. (2001). *The essential Drucker*. New York: HarperCollins.
2. Csikszentmihalyi, M. (2003). *Good business: Leadership, flow, and the making of meaning*. New York: Penguin Putnam Books.
3. *Harvard Business Review*, Boston, MA.

4. Assaraf, J., & Smith, M. (2008). *The answer: Grow any business, achieve financial freedom, and live an extraordinary life.* New York: Atria Books.
5. Kaplan, R., & Norton, D. (1996). *The balanced scorecard: Translating strategy into action.* Boston: Harvard Business School Press.

REVIEW QUESTIONS

1. The remains of the oldest hospital date back to when?
2. What three reimbursement models have had significant impact in health care?
3. Which reimbursement model introduced health care to the DRG?
4. List three drivers responsible for increasing healthcare costs.
5. What is an actuary?
6. List an example of a for-profit, a government, and a not-for-profit healthcare provider.
7. Who are the two consumers of health care?

REFERENCES

Barakat, P. (2000, October–December). Paying the price of the BBA. *Business and Economic Review.* Retrieved April 7, 2009, from http://findarticles.com/p/articles/mi _qa5313/is_200010/ai_n21461425

Bureau of Labor Statistics (BLS). (2008). *Career Guide to Industries, 2008-09 edition.* Retrieved April 7, 2009, from http://www.bls.gov/oco/cg

Centers for Medicare and Medicaid Services (CMMS). (2008). *Key milestones in CMS programs.* Retrieved July 8, 2008, from http://www.cms.hhs.gov/History/Downloads/ CMSProgramKeyMilestones.pdf

Fetter, R. (2001). *A guide to the Robert Barclay Fetter Papers.* Manuscripts and Archives, Yale University Library. Retrieved July 9, 2008, from http://mssa.library.yale.edu/find aids/eadPDF/mssa.ms.1496.pdf

Harrington, C. (2007). How to improve nursing homes: One expert's 30-year view. *Aging Today, 28*(5). Retrieved July 8, 2008, from http://www.allhealth.org/BriefingMaterials/ AgingToday-Harrington-985.pdf

Kenny, J. (2008). *How to define business.* Retrieved July 21, 2008, from http://ezinearticles. com/?How-to-Define-a-Business&id=108146

Levit, K., Smith, C., Cowan, C., Lazenby, H., Sensenig, A., & Catlin, A. (2003). Trends in U.S. health care spending, 2001. *Health Affairs, 22*(1), 154–164.

Lynch, T. (1987). *Skating with Heather Grace.* Retrieved April 7, 2009, from http:// www.thomaslynch.com/skating.html (please visit Mr. Thomas's Web site for his collection of poetry)

Nagamine, H., Jaing, J., & Merrill, C. T. (2006). *Statistical Brief #14: Trends in elderly hospitalizations, 1997–2004.* Retrieved July 18, 2008, from http://www.ahrq.gov/data/hcup

National Coalition on Health Care. (2006). *Facts on health insurance coverage.* Retrieved July 10, 2008, from http://www.nchc.org/fact/coverage.shtml

Pear, R. (2002, February 12). 9 of 10 nursing homes in U.S. lack adequate staff, a government study finds. *The New York Times.* Retrieved April 7, 2009, from http://www.nytimes.com/2002/02/18/us/9-of-10-nursing-homes-in-us-lack-adequate-staff-a-government-study-finds.html?scp=1&sq=9%20of%2010%20nursing%20homes%20lack%20adequate%20staff,%20study%20finds&st=cse

Steuerle, E. (2007, October 8). Blurring the line between charities and businesses. *Washington Post,* p. D03. Retrieved April 7, 2009, from http://www.washingtonpost.com/wp-dyn/content/article/2007/10/07/AR2007100701167.html

Stoil, M. J. (2001). *Will CMS be everyone's friend?* Retrieved May 1, 2009, from http://www.thefreelibrary.com/Will+CMS+Be+Everyone's+Friend%3f-a079355467

Taheri, P. A, Butz, D. A., & Greenfield, L. J. (2000). Length of stay has minimal impact on the cost of hospital admission. *Journal of the American College of Surgeons, 191*(2), 123–130. Retrieved July 14, 2008, from http://www.journalacs.org/article/S1072-7515(00)00352-5/fulltext

Thompson, T. (2002). *From diagnosis to payment: The dynamics of coding systems for hospital, physician, and other health services.* Prepared by K. Matherlee for the Secretary of the U.S. Department of Health and Human Services, National Health Policy Forum. Retrieved April 7, 2009, from http://www.nhpf.org/library/background-papers/BP_Coding_1-02.pdf

U.S. Census Bureau. (2004). *Population estimates.* Retrieved July 20, 2008, from http://www.census.gov/popest/estimates.php

Wall, J. K. (2007). *Senex grows as unpaid hospital bills take off.* Retrieved July 21, 2008, for http://www.redorbit.com/news/health

PART 2

The Principles and Foundations of Strategic Planning

CHAPTER 4

Just What Is Strategic Planning?

OBJECTIVES

1. Compare strategic planning to the nursing process.
2. Identify the components of strategic planning.
3. Recognize similarities between critical thinking and strategic thinking.
4. Differentiate between internal factors and external factors.
5. Explain what is meant by performance targets.
6. Review the three key components to a strategic plan.
7. Identify the stakeholders of strategic planning.
8. Clarify values and vision.
9. Differentiate between ordinary and strategic objectives.

Planning implies prioritizing tasks with available resources—business as usual. *Strategic* planning implies rethinking priority tasks with available resources to achieve a new business result. This chapter offers necessary vocabulary and lays the foundation for understanding the tenets of the strategic planning process. Key components and principles that lead to a successful strategic plan are introduced.

DEFINING STRATEGY, STRATEGIC PLANS, AND THE STRATEGIC PLANNING PROCESS: GETTING OVER JARGON INTIMIDATION

We have been nurses for a combined 49 years, and it was not until we had the privilege (and challenge) of innovating and implementing a complex educational initiative that we ran head-on into the realization—an epiphany—that nursing and nursing education do not always function smoothly when encountering change. Nursing, and many pockets of nursing education, does not operate from the principles and ethics of standard rules of business engagement. Nursing and nursing education do not operate smoothly within business process. The culture of nursing has created its own internal chasm between what we do and where we work. This chasm has led to ongoing disconnects that continue to fuel the nursing shortage and that are a primary reason that nurses are exiting the profession.

That makes sense; nurses provide care. As we've covered in Part 1, care and business operate from two distinct paradigms, and professionally, very different skill and knowledge sets are taught, practiced, and mastered. When we think back on all the frustrations, angst, and malcontent within our nursing careers, most have flowed from the fundamental disconnect between business and care. Once we recognized our professional omissions and gaps in knowledge, we set out to better understand what was missing, why nursing meetings were so exasperating, why administration did not "understand" or value our concerns, and how we could garner skills that facilitated change, innovation, and responsiveness: an empowered profession that reclaims and asserts the love of nursing. This text is the first step in helping other nurses to cross that very chasm and to help all nurses understand how to conceive, plan, and implement—or at the very least, function within—a strategic plan.

Before we launch into the tenets of strategic planning, we would like you to think about what you do every day in your nursing practice: the nursing process. Assessment, diagnosis, planning, implementation, and evaluation are the key ingredients of the practice of care. Sometimes the nursing process can seem uncompromising and tedious as we try to figure out which "related to" item of the North American Nursing Diagnosis Association—or any other nursing diagnostic terminology—would best be suited to our purpose of identifying and explaining our client's care needs. If we allow ourselves to become mired in the minutiae of terms and verbiage, it is very easy to become annoyed and ineffectively employ the very process that is meant to standardize professional nursing communication. Although we agree that the nursing language has become a little convoluted and esoteric, if we remember its purpose—effective communication and improved care outcomes—the process is pretty straightforward.

Strategic planning and the nursing process have a great deal in common; both seek improved outcomes, both can be simple, quick, and easily executed, both can become mired in jargon and esoterism, and both must be a part of daily decision-making and cultural expectation in order to accomplish their purpose: improved care. Instead of the eternal feeling of frustration, and sometimes helplessness and befuddlement, that we were constantly met with whenever we set out to implement, or were charged with, quality improvement, we are now empowered by the marriage of care and business. One does not negate the other; business skills strengthen our ability to provide and advocate for care.

Simply put, strategic planning involves these questions:

- Where are we?
- Where do we need and want to be?
- What is the best way to get there?
- How do we evaluate our progress?

An understanding of the strategic planning process lays the groundwork necessary for participating in quality improvement, change, and innovation. It is a common-sense tool that illuminates the "yellow brick road" to whatever your or your organization's definition of an emerald city may be. So, here we go with some definitions as we embark on the journey of strategic planning— which is just planning with a clear vision and a structured format—one that assesses and defines specific pieces of the planning process and that creates the roadmap from today's vision to tomorrow's reality.

Glossary of Terms

Strategic planning: "The objective of strategic planning is to develop a practical tool that can guide an organization into some defined future and provide important measures of success" (Burns, 1994, pg. 1). It is a written outline of the future that should enhance efficiency and effectiveness, encourage unity and focus, empower meaningful change, and streamline decision-making— succinctly, magnificently intelligent resource management.

Strategic plan: Planned change or a roadmap of how to get from where you are to where you want to be. This is the "how do we get there?" piece, just like the map in your car's glove box. It is based on a set of goals and objectives that help you or your organization move forward. This plan differentiates an enterprise and gives it competitive advantage (improved quality or capacity). Strategic plans weigh all variables and determine the "best" direction.

Example of a strategic plan: a plan that intentionally drives your ideas, your practice, your organization, or your business forward. For our following examples, we will develop a plan to educate and train nurses in the principles of care and business while considering the multitude of influences. It can be as simple as a plan to be accepted into a nursing program, or as complicated as a plan to redesign a nursing curriculum.

Please think about a strategic plan that you have developed and implemented in the past:

Strategy: *Action steps* to get from where you are today to your envisioned future, and being clear about where you are going and why—based on today's healthcare arena and the arena of the future (these action steps are called strategies and direct your mission in the best possible direction).

Example of a strategy: (1) Secure a book contract. (2) Write a book on strategic planning as a foundational strategy to assist nurses to better understand the synergy that can be created between principles of business and care.

Please think about a strategy that would help you to take action on your vision and mission:

Strategic planning process: This is the "prestrategic" planning piece, not unlike the assessment and diagnostic pieces to the NP. This is a coordinated and systematic process that lays the framework for how the plan will proceed—the direction of the plan that will best optimize the future outcomes (responsive to dynamic environments). The strategic planning process is also referred to as *strategic review.*

Example of the strategic planning (*review*) process: We identified a need, defined our vision and mission, and brainstormed the many ways (strategies) that we could get from where we were to where we wanted to be. There were many perspectives and methods that we could have thought about employing to accomplish our purpose (such as peace and possibility for the world's children, created by nursing's actualization of its highest vision of care), but we needed to choose the best process for us based on who we are, our likes and dislikes, our talents and abilities, etc. (our "culture"). For us, that plan involved four distinct components: authoring, a Web-based business, training, and consulting. You can see that each of these components requires an overall strategic plan and individual plans and strategies if we are to implement them successfully and sustainably.

Please think about what components your strategic plan will need in order to actualize your personal or professional purpose:

Strategic thinking: "It has always been done that way" is the antithesis of strategic thinking. We call it *critical thinking*—a buzzword for using your cranial matter. But it is more than that; critical thinking and strategic thinking are based on principles of inquiry, evidence, creativity, open-mindedness, acceptance of diversity, and truth-seeking (learning). Strategic thinking has three key components.

> Three key components of strategic thinking:
>
> 1. The vision (and developing that vision)
> 2. Wisdom (clear and cultural "knowing" of your profession/business and all the players and variables that affect that profession/business)
> 3. Creative problem-solving (based on the vision and sound judgment, effective solutions are created; "thinking outside the box"—or, as Dr. Covey (1992) would say, "a break with"—may be the best solution).

A popular expression is, "nothing fails like success." In other words, "it has always been done that way" may have worked last week or last year, but there are now new challenges; we may have new evidence and learning, or we may have discovered a better way to accomplish our work. It is time to rethink, problem-solve, and create better solutions based on what we know today and what our best intelligent "guess" projection will be for tomorrow, next month, and 5 years from now. Our favorite synonym for strategic is "responsive."

Example of strategic thinking: Our vision—peace and possibility for the world's children, created by nurses' actualization of their highest vision of care. Our "wisdom"—49 years in nursing and continual learning; creative problem-solving; stepping a little outside the "regular" nursing text box and trying to look at nursing's dilemmas through new lenses.

Please think about how you employ and resist strategic thinking and how strategic thinking is or is not employed by your organization. Conversely, have you resisted or not employed strategic thinking in your organization?

_____

_____

Strategy engineer: This is the liaison who tracks the plan's progress, tends to the organizing and planning, and communicates with all stakeholders about goals and the action steps to accomplish those goals, focusing on the objectives within each goal. One pitfall of any planning process is the omission of this key role. Someone has to be sure that the plan is not put on a shelf, only to be dusted off at next year's staff meeting. Have you ever taken part in a planning process—all creativity and enthusiasm for positive change—only to forget about it the minute the day-to-day work resumed?

Values: Principles, priorities, and standards that drive thought, action, and attitudes.

Examples of values: Empowered nursing, integrity, respect for others, cultural acceptance, peace, childhood for every child, and excellence.

Please list your three top values:

_____

_____

Vision: Imaginative insight and foresight (envisioned future) based on values (this is also sometimes referred to as your purpose—the "why we are here" piece).

Examples of vision: Peace and possibility for the world's children, created by nurses' actualization of their highest vision of care.

Please think about your vision for nursing and for your career as a nurse:

_____

_____

Mission: Tasks or goals assumed based on values and vision (tasks or goals to actualize the expressed values and vision).

Example of mission statements:

1. Educate and train nurses to be clear about "why we are here"— because we care.
2. Educate and train nurses in the tenets of business.

Please think of one mission that would lead to the actualization of your vision:

_____

_____

Continual improvement: Whenever we think about quality indicators or improving anything, we must first have a reference point of something that needs to be improved. Similar to the evaluation of the nursing process, nurses are constantly evaluating whether the therapies implemented are working, and without realizing it, we are constantly looking to improve care to obtain the desired outcomes. We know that there are errors in patient care when a medication is incorrectly administered, hence the need for quality improvement. It does not matter if we call it continuous quality improvement (CQI), quality improvement (QI), total quality improvement (TQI), continual improvement (CI), or any other acronym or abbreviation; we identify that a problem exists and find a way to make "it" better. It is a continual process.

Example of CI: Identifying the chasm between principles of care and business. We recognize the need to implement a CI initiative.

Please think about how you might apply the concept of CI to the area that you have identified as needing improvement:

_____

_____

Time frame: A strategic plan describes where a person (personal strategic plan), organization, or business is going over a set period of time. Depending on the need and problems identified, the strategic plan may be for 6 months, 1 year, or 5 or more years. Many plans incorporate both short-term and long-range plans and the strategies necessary to get there.

Example of a time frame: Short-term: Submit completed application to nursing program by deadline. Long-term: Complete program within 4 years.

Please think about the time frame necessary to solve the problem that you have identified:

Short-term:

_____

_____

Long-term:

_____

_____

Long-range planning versus strategic planning: This is a point for clarification. Long-range planning is used to set a goal over a "long" period of time—often several years. For example, in 10 years, I will pay off my school loans and save for a new car. Strategic planning, on the other hand, helps me not only to calculate how I will pay off my school loans and which car I will buy but also to determine the best strategies to help me get there and to identify and anticipate all the variables that will affect that goal and how to deal with them.

Situational analysis: Here is where individuals or organizations take a hard look at *where they are* in relation to *where they want to be* and in relation to the world around them—taking stock. This piece of the strategic planning process takes a look at the *background*—why you are where you are—and a look at current realities and determines the ideal "next" (part of the strategic review).

Example of a situation analysis: A nurse currently holds an associate degree in nursing and recognizes the limited opportunities for career advancement; consider all relevant factors affecting current job opportunities.

Please think about a current personal or professional situation, and conduct a situational analysis (where have you been, where are you, and where do you want to go?):

_____

_____

Competitive advantage: What sets you or your organization apart from others? Obviously, you want quality in whatever you are doing to be cardinal; care, after all, is not like Wal-Mart, whose slogan is "save money, live better" (although there may be a hospital CEO or two who likes this slogan). This is also called "market niche"; what do you (or your organization) do that is unique, or better than or unequaled by anyone else? Some hospitals are the baby hospitals or the heart centers. This is not happenstance; they have strategically identified a need and gone after that market share (yes, we know, it's a little harsh to think about capturing baby market shares, but that is today's reality). Also, please recall the branding of the Magnet Recognition Program and why hospitals seek that designation.

Example of competitive advantage: We identified that few are discussing the gap in care as an expression of empowered synergy. Strengthening nursing— care—by strengthening nursing's role in business processes across all levels of nursing is not just for advanced practice and management anymore.

Please think about how you or your organization might create a competitive edge (advantage) over your "competitors" (in the friendliest sense):

Internal factors ("environment"): This is where you identify your or your organization's strengths and weaknesses. These come in many "resource" forms: financial (Do you have enough money? Can you get enough, and can you optimally manage the money?), facility (like office space, equipment, location, and even how to heat the building), human (enough people, the right talents and abilities, ways to manage those valuable people, etc.), policies and procedures (Are you starting from scratch? Does everyone know the who, what, and why?), and the biggie, time (time management, enough time). Strengths and weaknesses are the first two components of a SWOT analysis (strengths, weaknesses, opportunities, and threats).

Example of internal factors: Financial. Authoring is a time commitment and does not require a large financial commitment. Facility: We have the necessary space and equipment to author. Human: We are maximizing our unique abilities and talents in the coauthoring process. Policy and procedure: We have identified and agreed on the necessary procedures and "policies" that guide our writing. Time: We have established a writing schedule but recognize the challenge of time management.

Please conduct a mini-assessment of what you see as your strengths and weaknesses, using the components just mentioned (financial, facility, human, policy/procedure, and time):

_____

_____

External factors or "environment": These are influences outside your or your organization's sphere of influence—these are *opportunities* and *threats* (the last two pieces of the SWOT analysis). Opportunities are areas for growth, unclaimed market share, or identification of a problem and creation of a viable solution. Threats can be decreased Medicare reimbursement, regulations that inhibit or restrict solutions, others' competition and market saturation (too much product and not enough buyers), economic drivers, etc.

Example of external factors: Opportunities: Schools of nurses are in demand and the need is projected to grow. The nursing shortage and worldwide workforce crisis will continue to require professionally trained nurses. Threats: More attractive career options for women, non-competitive wages, difficult work with long shifts, job hazards—such as risk of back injuries and infectious diseases—and variable work hours.

Please think about what opportunities and threats exist for your idea for a strategic plan:

_____

_____

SWOT Analysis: Just a recap: SWOT stands for strengths, weaknesses, opportunities, and threats (see Appendix 4a: SWOT Worksheet).

Balanced Scorecard: We can thank two Harvard professors—Robert S. Kaplan and David P. Norton—for this tool, which helps corral the constituent parts of the strategic planning process. The purpose of the Balanced Scorecard is to help managers and leaders to mobilize the necessary resources to effect change on the path to the company's vision. "Managers, like pilots, need instrumentation about many aspects of their environment and performance to monitor the journey toward excellent future outcomes" (Kaplan & Norton, 1996, p. 2). We will take a closer look at the Balanced Scorecard in Chapter 9 and basically show you how to employ this process tool. We are sure that your administration has a clear understanding of this tool, and most likely, your work and work environment are influenced by Kaplan and Norton's work.

Market focus: This is all about focusing on your customers. Imagine opening a clinic in a retirement community that focuses on well-baby care. Having a clearer market focus, a preventive health clinic that offers a specialty in gerontology would be more appropriate.

Example of a market-focused business: As we write this text, we continually think of being in a room with nurses, average age 47, 93% female, 85% of whom work in a hospital, etc., and the dilemmas facing "every nurse." We draw from our years of experience in nursing across the spectrum of care. We are also acutely aware of the many ways and places that nurses practice care, and we continually try to respect care across all levels and disciplines.

Please think about the market focus that you or your organization has or wants to capture:

Performance targets: Nursing may be more familiar with the term outcome measures, but the bottom line with both is that you cannot reach a goal (target) if it is not clearly defined and measurable. The CMS has set the "never events"—clear, measurable outcomes that will never happen (or at least, never be reimbursed for by CMS). Negative goals are one way to set performance targets or outcome measures, but they are hard to measure, just like the effectiveness of prevention is hard to quantify. Performance targets are easiest to work with when

In its position statement, *Innovation in Nursing Education: A Call to Reform*, the National League for Nursing (NLN) has challenged the way "it [nursing education] has always been done": "What is needed now is dramatic reform and innovation in nursing education to create and shape the future of nursing practice" (NLN, 2005). The NLN has set out 11 recommendations to create the new future for nursing education and nursing (please visit the NLN's Web site at http://www.nln.org). The performance targets that the NLN has set are innovation and dramatic reform based on sound pedagological models and research—pretty encompassing and complex targets that require sound strategic thinking and the ability of nursing educators and stakeholders to strategically plan.

they are tangible. Tangible targets in business are often related to profit hallmarks; reach 1 million in revenues or sell 5 million hamburgers.

Please think about which performance measures you are held to and what your work unit is expected to achieve:

_____

_____

Contingency plan: Any plan of value must be dynamic, but plans must also have "rainy day" clauses and be flexible. Contingency plans fall under three types:

1. Planning for unforeseen consequences: Planning for unforeseen and usually uncontrollable events. For example, employees can get the flu, stock markets will fluctuate, and hurricanes do come ashore. Of course, no one can prepare for every eventuality, but a good plan recognizes the need for a continuity of operations plan.
2. Risk evaluation: Evaluate and plan for the risks that affect a business/profession (e.g., sufficient capital [money] to pay for repairs, upgrades).
3. Disasters: Plan for disasters, such as what to do when capacities are reached or mass casualties occur, regardless of etiology.

All three are contingency plans that should be addressed within a strategic plan.

These definitions and examples are the big picture of strategic planning. We have included a detailed glossary in Appendix 4b.

WHAT ARE THE COMPONENTS OF A STRATEGIC PLAN?

Strategic plans can be mammoth documents (think of the nation's disaster plan), or they can be one-page narratives that help you to decide which emergency phone numbers you want to program into your home phone. Regardless of the size and scope of a strategic plan, they all have three key areas—pieces of the process puzzle of strategic planning. Again, you will recognize the similarity to the NP.

Assessment: Taking Stock, Strategic Review

The first step in any change process is to do a "quick check" to determine organizational or personal fit. Before time and money are spent, ideas need to pass through a simple process that checks any change against the four criteria illustrated in Figure 4-1.

The three key components of a strategic plan are:

1. Assessment—take stock and determine fit (whether the plan is right for us now): *Strategic Review*

2. Set direction, and refine and adopt (the plan): *Clarifying Values and Vision* (akin to the diagnosis process)

3. Implement and evaluate: *Strategic Objectives* (akin to planning, implementation, and evaluation in the NP)

Figure 4-1 Quick check.

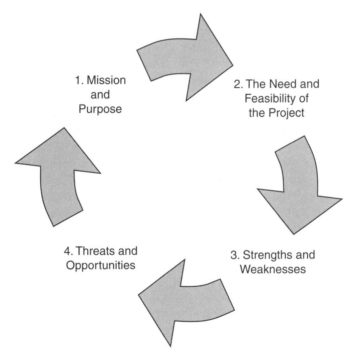

1. Mission and Purpose
2. The Need and Feasibility of the Project
3. Strengths and Weaknesses
4. Threats and Opportunities

1. Is the change in alignment with the enterprise's purpose and mission?
2. Is the need clearly identified and feasible?
3. Do the strengths outweigh the weaknesses?
4. Do the opportunities outweigh the threats?

This quick check can weed out both obvious and not so obvious misfits for an organization; we are sure that we can think of many "miss-guided" managers who led us off on projects that were not relevant and, perhaps more commonly, who failed to take action on necessary directions. If the purpose is education, an innovation for a better shoelace may not be an appropriate strategic direction. On the other hand, a better Web-based learning system may be an essential strategy worth pursuing, both for the benefit of the learner and for the strategic positioning of the educational institution.

Quick checks are not meant to deter strategic planning (planned change); it might very well be that planned change is exactly what is needed. The purpose and mission may be outdated or no longer responsive to today's healthcare arena; weakness may seem to overshadow strengths, but perhaps external resources could be accessed that would tip that balance. Opportunities may become cardinal if the threats are so great that the enterprise may succumb without innovation. (A simple example of this is an overweight client with high blood pressure, diabetes mellitus, coronary vascular disease, and transient ischemic attacks; the patient has many threats and weaknesses, but opportunities for improved health could be captured by discovering the client's strengths and the strengths of his or her resource base. If something isn't done, a disastrous outcome is most likely.)

Ultimately, it is the leaders' responsibility to determine if there are sufficient resources to implement a strategic planning (change) process, the extent of that process, and the intent of the process. Lack of resources, failing systems, or any other business dysfunction by no means negate the need for a strategic plan. In fact, the necessity for a strategic plan is magnified when things are not going well. This quick check may serve to accentuate the need for a planning process. Another popular expression is appropriate here: "Insanity is doing the same thing over and over and expecting different results." Indeed, failing to recognize the need to embark on a strategic planning process is often far more detrimental than the resource challenges of embarking on the planning process.

After an initial quick check (something that we all hope our leaders do on a regular basis with many different elements) and the decision to undertake a strategic planning process, the assessment process must begin in earnest.

Think about what you do when you enter a client's room; you take in the big picture and notice everything from respiratory rates and audible breath sounds to IV pumps, skin color, lines, linens, light, visitors, body language, wound vacs, Foley drainage, and any number of other aspects that affect the well-being of the client. If you responded to an IV pump alarm but did not notice the profuse sanguineous drainage on the sheet, your assessment would be incomplete and could lead to dire consequences for the client. All assessments are virtually the same; they must be thorough to be of any value.

Once the leadership (or you, as your own leader in a personal strategic plan) has determined the need to implement a strategic plan, a more detailed assessment process begins: the strategic review. This is a tough process; think of it as a total-body scan. Everything is laid open for review, and many eyes will see the internal workings of the business. How would you feel if, right now, several other people had full access to your finances? They get to look at your credit habits and history, see how you balance your checkbook, see how much you spent on that frilly underwear—everything. And then they will get out a calculator and analyze it—the good, the bad, and the ugly. In health care, we often "discover" or validate areas that need improvement through quality assurance initiatives that begin with thorough assessment.

This effort requires a high level of professional and personal maturity and accountability. The other vital piece to an all-encompassing assessment process is that of sensitive and compassionate leadership. In health care, many have been on the receiving end of an accreditation process or an employee evaluation review that has been punitive and demeaning. Little in the way of improvement or corrective action ever comes from such unenlightened "management" practice; often, the bad results are perpetuated or soon resurface. We don't assess a patient by tossing him or her to and fro at our discretion; the patient is handled with respect, human kindness, and professionalism that are based on knowledge and understanding. The strategic review (assessment) must be handled with the same qualities.

A WORD OF WARNING

The strategic review is a crucial piece that can inadvertently render the strategic plan futile if it purposely or inadvertently exacerbates a dysfunction that might otherwise remain innocuous. Imagine an overworked middle manager who knows that his budgets are not complete, whose filing is 2 months behind, who has policies piled on the corner of his desk, and whose new administrator expects him to be a team player and work as long as the job requires. Now, with the strategic review process, everything will be open to scrutiny and judgment. Can you see how strategic plans may meet undue resistance, or not even get off the ground because of a lack of sensitivity to system, workgroup, or individual dysfunction? This is a potentially touchy process; please tread respectfully.

Please think about a review process that laid blame or focused solely on what wasn't working. What was the consequence—was there lasting improvement?

Example: A strategic plan is begun to decrease hospital-wide medication errors. As a tool to deter medication errors, the unit manager places a poster with individual nurses' names and any medication errors they are suspected of making—highlighted in red—at the nurses' station.

Our professional work can be just as hallowed as our personal matters, and perhaps more so if egos are actively engaged. Another word of warning about beginning a strategic review: Attempting change in a business culture that is dogmatic, punitive, or autocratic is very difficult and may lead to excessive head-banging behaviors. You have three options when working in such a culture:

1. You must go into a change/improvement endeavor with patience, an attitude of inquiry, and fortitude.
2. Find a work environment that is conducive to positive change.
3. Forget about improvement processes, and grin and bear it.

The strategic review is much like assessing your personal finances. You can keep writing checks and charging more items, and hope that everything will be OK. However, assessing spending patterns, budgeting, planning, and figuring out the best strategies to achieve financial success will better contribute to the attainment of financial well-being. However painful and tedious a strategic review may be, knowledge and the truth about an enterprise are far more valuable than glossed-over views or polite dismissals of dysfunction. Whenever you hold something up to the light, please be sensitive to what may be exposed and to the people who may have their professional souls on the line. It may be those very dysfunctions that need resolution—or extraction—to facilitate positive growth. Respect people first, processes second; for processes are nothing without the people to implement them.

Clarifying Values and Vision

Have you ever worked in a hospital or other healthcare facility and been asked to function in what felt like a conflict of values? Perhaps you value quality patient care (yes, we know that you do) but are asked to care for and supervise 10 postoperative (let's say all post–major gastrointestinal surgery) clients. You would do your very best, but the incongruence between what you value and your work reality is a powerful example of how we, as nurses, can be led away from our core values and those of our facilities. In fact, we venture to assert that most discontent in the nurse's work environment stems from a clash in values. In a Canadian study, 74% of all workers said that it is important to work for employers whose values are in line with their own (Foord Kirk, 2008).

Values are nonnegotiable; they evolve from learning, intellectual inquiry, culture and belief systems, and social influences. Personal and social values are not static. In 1880, reading, writing, arithmetic, and industry were values in elementary education, whereas the core values of elementary education in 2008 may encompass cultural tolerance, art appreciation, and personal empowerment. Values are deeply personal while simultaneously being deeply embedded in the current culture. We asked you to think about your values in Chapter 2 and earlier in this chapter. We would like you to answer a couple of simple questions here: Are your values in alignment with those of your place of employment, and visa versa? If you answered "no" to either of these questions, are you considering, or have you considered, leaving your position?

It has been interesting, over the path of our nursing careers, to note how many of our colleagues cannot state their values. We have asked you a few times now to think about and state your values. "To thine own self be true"; if you have not deeply thought about "who" you are, it is very likely that you can be led in many directions. It is not that you do not have deeply felt values; it is often that we were never taught to think about, question, and assert those values. We imagine that you have many little quirks that have never been held up to the light because they are "just you." Think not only what your values are but why you hold those values and how you express them in your life.

Here is an analogy about why we need to question "what always has been based on what we believe (value)" and why we believe what we do. Suzie was preparing a ham to cook for dinner and cut off the end before putting it in the roaster. Her son asked, "Why do you do that?" Suzie wasn't sure, but she knew that's how you were supposed to cook a ham. Curious, she called her mother and asked why a ham had to be cut and cooked that way. Her mom said, "Because that is how to cook a ham." Suzie's mom then got curious and called her mother: "Why do we cut the end off of a ham before cooking?" Her mother said, "Because the roasting pan is too small." Make sure that you are not operating from the paradigm that your roasting pan is too small!

Continuing with this analogy, let's say that Suzie has inherited her grandmother's roasting pan and takes a cooking class from Julia Child that firmly advocates no ham cutting before roasting. After her class, she goes home. She has the same roasting pan but now she has to work with a noncut ham; her ham won't fit. Everything she now knows does not fit with what she once held as reality—using her grandmother's roasting pan, she would first cut off the end of the ham. She has new knowledge that does not fit her old circumstances. She has two choices: keep cutting her ham even though it will dry out and get tough (poor patient outcomes), or get a new roasting pan (expand her abilities and acquire new or strengthened values). We want to suggest that getting a smaller ham is not a solution in this analogy; we can't shrink our patients. New learning often renders old values obsolete—hence, the need for lifelong learning. We need to keep fresh eyes on our world "hams," professionally and personally.

We have illustrated the importance of identifying and adhering to core values (core values are those values from which all others flow; if your core value is family, then values of respect, kindness, encouragement, etc., would naturally flow from that one core value). Setting direction—whether it is for a family, a ham, a group, or a business—requires that everything begin with articulating, understanding, and accepting core values. If just one concept in strategic planning could be learned from this text, it is this: Regardless of the endeavor, everyone must understand, believe in, and agree to the cornerstone—the quoin that supports everything else: values. Values are the standards by which every task, every goal, and every accomplishment is measured.

Vision comes easily once values are clearly stated. Discovering and uncovering values shines a light on what previously was hidden. Vision is the natural outflow of values. Do you know the values for your place of employment? Is there a separate set of values for the floor or unit that you work on? Have you or your family discussed and written your values?

Do you have a personal vision—an ideal—of what you'd like your life to be, including everything from every domain (from family, love, and friends to recreation, money, home, spirit, and education)? Developing a vision for an enterprise is like defining your ideal life. In business terms, a vision includes the ideal customer, net profits, ideal location, ideal employee, ideal market position (e.g., "No. 1 heart hospital"), ideal outcomes (based on regulations, standards, evidence-based practice [EBP], benchmarks, ethics, and guidelines), ideal culture and attitudes, etc. Is your personal vision for your professional life in harmony with your organization's vision? Take a minute or longer to answer why or why not; you don't want to be cutting off the end of your ham for irrelevant reasons.

Strategic Objectives

Strategic objectives correspond to the nursing processes' planning, implementation, and evaluation phases. After taking a hard look at current realities (assessment) and being clear about the ideal outcome (diagnosis), it is time to close the gap between the where-we-are-now and the where-we-want-to-be pieces. This is the how-to phase—how to get from where we are to where we want to be. These are no ordinary objectives; these are strategic objectives. There may be many paths (objectives) that lead to a preferred destination, but a strategic planning process captures the most efficient and beneficial paths and optimizes use of available resources; they are strategic—strategic objectives.

How can you tell when an objective is ordinary and when one is strategic? Think about our nursing process correlation. A patient has a fever of 103.5°F. She is not at a good place; you want her to be at 101°F or lower. You can create many objectives (paths) that may lead to decreased body temperature: (1) create a cool environment, to 35°F; (2) create an internal temperature of 98.8°F by administering ice water peritoneal lavage; or (3) administer prescribed antipyretics, remove linens and excess clothing, apply a cool sponge bath, and treat the underlying cause. Strategic objectives are the smartest (EBP), quickest, and safest ways to get you or your organization from where you are to where you want to be. (We hope that you chose Option 3 as the most strategic.)

With our patient example, we determined the best plan to reduce her fever, and then we implemented that plan. In nursing, it is obvious what we do next: We make sure that the plan and implementation (treatment) worked, and we evaluate the effectiveness of our plan and implementation by reassessing the patient's temperature. Strategic objectives are evaluated in much the same way.

To determine the success of an enterprise's strategic objectives (based, of course, on the expressed values and vision), we establish measurement criteria. Strategic objectives may be measured at intervals, sometimes referred to as hallmarks, milestones, or sentinel events (sentinel events are also markers of quality). For our patient, a hallmark may be a temperature of 102.5°F within 1 hour—not there yet, but on the right path. So, strategic objectives are twofold: They are the *best route* to take, and they are *measurable*. Hallmarks and sentinel events can be marked along the path to determine if the project—the strategies identified and employed—is indeed leading to the desired outcome.

WHO NEEDS TO BE INVOLVED WITH A STRATEGIC PLAN?

Before others are asked to participate, a strategic planning team must be organized. This team will sponsor and facilitate the strategic planning project. This team then needs to determine workgroups. At the foundation of the *who* is assuring some level of readiness. Does management support the change? Is there a board or other directors who must support the project? Do we have sufficient resources to undertake a strategic planning process? Are we in crisis?

Is this the right time for a strategic planning project? How willing is the culture to embrace change? It is possible that pretraining and education must occur before a strategic planning project can be implemented?

Strategic plans must include everyone whom the strategic plan affects or will affect. This may be a tall order, so let's take a look at what this means. Strategic plans may be unit specific (to increase client satisfaction 50% on the medical-surgical floor), they may be facility-wide (e.g., become the telemedicine center for the Northwest), or they may be limited to a facility-wide discipline (e.g., 90% retention and 100% expressed job satisfaction for housekeeping staff). In each instance, a competitive edge is being sought.

In these examples, there are some obvious actors who must be included in the strategic planning process of strategic review, clarifying values and vision, and setting strategic objectives. On the other hand, not everyone needs to be, or realistically can be, involved in all three phases. The strategic review is often completed by management under the direction of leadership. Needs are discovered through quality indicators or quality assessment processes. Strategic review, then, is most often the domain of leaders and managers. That isn't to say that a grassroots strategic review is not equally valuable; sometimes the staff identify and understand a problem, need, or direction better than management or leadership.

A poor management practice is to get staff fired up, empower a vision process, ask people to work hard and contribute to the vision and mission, and then wait until the next annual all-staff meeting to tell them what has or has not been done with their valuable professional creativity and work; they will have forgotten, and/or they may feel betrayed. If staff are asked to be engaged in a heart- and intellect-searching process, they must be honored for their contribution. Ideas are often personal expressions, and individuals become vested in those ideas. When an employee is vested, he or she will be more productive, buy in to the change process, and be happier with the workplace. Be sure to respect those whom you ask for input, and be sure that you understand their "reward" (whether it be further participation, specific roles, or published credit).

The stage at which the strategic planning process needs to begin determines who needs to be involved. If staff will only meet annually to work on redefining the vision and mission, they must be kept appraised throughout the year. A fundamental principle of working with adults is that they will learn, participate, and contribute if they understand the value in what is at hand. Recall the key role of the strategy liaison.

Let's say that a hospital nursing staff of 100 nurses are asked to help delineate the vision and mission to create a premier 21st-century medical-surgical facility. A total of 100 nurses (or 100 of any professional discipline) working on a strategic plan would be an unwieldy proposition—when they could all meet, what room would be large enough, who would pay for refreshments, how consensus would be built, who would be in charge and why, who would cover the floor, how the night shift would participate and so on. It may be important to involve all 100 in the vision and mission, but the process would be too cumbersome to carry through every strategic planning phase and meeting. Here is where the strategic engineer is crucial. Without a liaison who connects the project with all of the stakeholders, a change process may be doomed—or, at the very least, excruciatingly painful. The strategic engineer, for example, may determine that individual nursing units will meet monthly; housekeeping will meet every 2 months; dietary will not be involved until midproject or after the assessment is completed—you get the picture.

Identifying all stakeholders, determining the phase or component of the strategic plan in which the stakeholders will be of most value, deciding which piece stakeholders will need to be vested in, and deciding how each stakeholder will be included in the planning process are key leadership and management decisions that must be addressed in the strategic review. Overlooking or minimizing staff involvement can work, but that would be a 20th-century "industrial" paradigm that disrespects the knowledge worker of the 21st century. Each stage of the process will need to involve various people and groups at different times. Nursing is about people and care. By definition, nurses thrive on involvement; the more nurses are involved in this process, the richer and more comprehensive the plan will be.

PROJECT VERSUS TECHNICAL STRATEGIES

There are some key differences between project strategies and technical strategies; basically, one is encompassing, and one is more circumscribed. The strategic plan has outlined that the vision is to become a premier medical-surgical hospital. A project strategy is one that sets a direction: Hospital A will achieve Magnet Status by 2010 as part of the vision of becoming a premier medical-surgical hospital. A technical strategy would be to implement electronic medical records hospital-wide as a part of the vision of becoming a premier medical-surgical hospital. A project strategy is more "global" in its scope, whereas a technical strategy is more like a building block that enables other project components. Technical strategies do not necessarily involve technology; these strategies address infrastructure, whereas project strategies address a larger framework of standards or a target capacity.

Another way to view project versus technical strategies is to think of project strategies as the art and science of managing a project, and technical strategies as solving technical problems. Imagine that you need to plan a conference for 500 nurses. Project strategies would involve marketing, facility management, designing the agenda and curriculum, etc. Technical strategies would involve knowing where the fire extinguishers are located and how to use them, where AV feeds are, and who the IT contact will be. Project strategies are the big view, and technical strategies are the pieces of the project.

If you work in information technology (IT), this definition may be more literal. Project strategies apply to any strategy necessary to complete a plan, and technical strategies apply to anything that involves a technology. Either way, one seeks to define steps in the big picture, and one defines smaller specific steps.

STRATEGIC THINKING AND "VISIONING": THE THINKS YOU CAN THINK!

Strategic thinking is not unlike critical thinking. Both require a sound knowledge of EBP, both require an attitude of inquiry, and both require a passion for learning, tolerance, and understanding. Like critical thinking, strategic thinking can be learned. The foundational piece of both is that critical and strategic thinking must be based on knowledge; those engaged in strategic thinking must have correct data and information. If we "found" 10 nurses who had been marooned on a desert island for the past 20 years and then asked them to really think about the best direction for a medical-surgical unit, they would not have sufficient knowledge to strategically think about the best solutions.

Some people simply cannot, or do not want to, engage in imaginative thinking; for their personal reasons, they may not feel comfortable expressing their views, or they may never have learned how. To facilitate and encourage strategic thinking, safe cultures that value ideas and their expression must either already exist or be created. Brainstorming is an effective tool to initiate strategic thinking but can only be effective in tolerant and encouraging environments. The strategic thinking process requires out-of-the-box thinking. All angles need to be examined—no rock left unturned—and inquiring minds will want to know all they can to make the best decisions.

THE VISIONING PROCESS . . . WHO?

Visioning isn't for everyone. Some people are linear thinkers, some are concrete thinkers, and some prefer the "colors" black and white. Visioning is a leap from where something is to where it may be. It is hard to get a horse to go into a chute if he cannot see beyond the chute. When it comes to being led through a visioning process, people are not all that different. Most of us want to see what is on the other side; we want to know how it relates to us and what the benefit will be. Creating a vision and a mission statement for the exercise of creating them—because "we should have a vision and mission statement"—is a poor justification; not unlike the horse that may bolt at entering a blind chute, people must see the value on the other side of a visioning process.

Visions based on core values determine strategic direction. Vision statements that sit on a shelf are meaningless and useless. For a vision to be relevant and worthwhile, it must be an active part of every employee's belief about his or her work. The cultural adoption of the vision of achieving Magnet Status by 2012 would require that every patient interaction, every evaluation, and every managerial decision be tied to one of the Magnet criteria. As the hospital strove to be recognized as a Magnet facility, not every employee would need to participate in the visioning process, but every employee would need to clearly see and believe in the vision; all must buy in to and work toward the same purpose.

REVIEW QUESTIONS

1. List three similarities between the nursing process and strategic planning.
2. What is the difference between a strategic plan and a strategy?
3. List the three key components of strategic thinking.
4. The strategic planning process is similar to what part(s) of the nursing process?
5. List two similarities and two differences between values and vision.
6. What is the difference between project and technical strategies?

REFERENCES

Burns, M. (1994). *Off the shelf: How to ensure that your strategic plan becomes a valued tool.* Branford, CT: Brody Weiser Burns.

Covey, S. R. (1992). *Principle centered leadership.* New York: Simon & Schuster.

Foord Kirk, J. (2008, January 21). "Report card" shows employer grades declining. *Toronto Star.* Retrieved September 26, 2008, from http://www.workopolis.com

Kaplan, R., & Norton, D. (1996). *The Balanced Scorecard: Translating strategy into action.* Boston: Harvard Business School Press.

National League for Nursing (NLN). (2005). *Position statement: Transforming nursing education.* Retrieved August 20, 2008, from http://www.nln.org/aboutnln/PositionStatements/transforming052005.pdf

SWOT Worksheet

SWOT Worksheet

Rate each item from 1 to 5: 1 = *not significant*; 2 = *some significance*;
3 = *significant*; 4 = *moderately high significance*; 5 = *very significant*

Strength	Rate (1–5)	Weakness	Rate (1–5)	Opportunities	Rate (1–5)	Threats	Rate (1–5)

SWOT Scorecard Worksheet

SWOT Item	Rating Total
Strength	
Weakness	
Opportunities	
Threats	
Decision	

Note: These are sample templates for a simple SWOT analysis. The worksheets can be expanded to include more variables or to assign timelines.

Glossary

Action plan—document that outlines the strategic objectives with the clear steps necessary for their achievement; may be called the operating plan

Action steps—the "who does what, when, and how" necessary to get the job done; are specific; job descriptions/tasks list

Alignment—everything "fits" with the overall purpose: infrastructure systems, outside support systems, people skills, attitudes, and talents—all resources—work to support the strategic goals

Bandwagon effect—people do things and believe things because others do (herding effect, lemming effect, etc.)

Benchmarking—comparison of a quality, achievement, or process against "the best" in the business; a self-evaluation tool

Business model—describes an enterprise's ability to generate income, what affects its revenue streams, the size of investment necessary, how success will be defined, and how each component interdependently functions

Core competency—the knowledge or skills that are essential to the key areas necessary to produce superlative services or products

Culture—an enterprise's values, habits, rituals/traditions, and operating form and style

Differentiation strategy—"set apart"; purposefully making the service or product distinctly different from others in the same market

Equity—value of shares issued by a company, or values of property minus the debt

Hurdle rate—a calculation on the rate of return on new projects; expected hurdle of increased cost with some time lag before profit is realized

Interlock—necessary collaboration to complete a goal

Judo strategy—strategic "moves" based on principles of movement, balance, and leverage (please see *Judo Strategy: Turning Your Competitor's Strength to Your Advantage*, David B. Yoffie and Mary Kwak, 1994)

Kaizen (improvement)—a Japanese business philosophy of continuous quality improvement wherein every employee is involved in the process and each contributes ideas and solutions; improvement as a way of life (may be referred to as "catch-ball," to play catch—everyone must be equally equipped as ideas and leadership are "tossed" among all "players")

Lead users—people or enterprises whose needs exceed those of "typical" users

Market segmentation—large customer aggregates are divided into smaller aggregate categories with more specific needs

Network congestion—too many users clog the system (as in traffic congestion or network congestion)

Network effect (externality)—a phenomenon created when more users exponentially create more value (as with cell phones; the existence of more cell phone users makes the cell phone more valuable to its user)

Operating margin—earnings before interest and taxes (EBIT) divided by net sales; used to determine profitability

Operating plan—physical necessities of your business's operation; physical location, facilities and equipment, inventory requirements and suppliers, a description of the manufacturing/product process, outline of the capital and expense—requirements for your business to operate from day to day

Positive feedback loop—perturbation that leads to perturbation in the same direction (means "throw into confusion/disturb," and that confusion/disruption creates more of the same—for example, diabetics crave sugar, sugar negatively alters the blood sugar, diabetics continue to crave sugar)

Price elasticity of demand (PED) (versus inelastic)—measurement of the consumer's price "sensitivity" ("elastic" refers to products/services that consumers are not likely to pay more for)

Process reengineering—breakthrough change based on reengineering—redesigning—processes (requires strategic thinking)

Return on assets (ROA)—net income divided by total assets

Return on equity (ROE)—measure of shareholder's stake; net income divided by shareholder's equity

Skunk works—a team assembled for the express purpose of generating innovation or to solve a particular problem; often conducted on a retreat or in an isolated setting to maximize focus (isn't this a great term!)

Substitute—a product or service that can fill the role of another; when an increase in the purchase of one is the consequence of the increased price of another (e.g., stents cost approximately one-third of the price of bypass surgery)

Work breakdown structure (WBS)—a tool that identifies the project's goals and breaks them down into tasks and subtasks necessary for the project's completion

CHAPTER 5

Tools from the Strategic Planning Workbench

──────── OBJECTIVES ────────

1. Identify the purpose and use of strategic maps.
2. Describe strategic intent.
3. Review unintended consequences.
4. Discuss force-field analysis, comparing positive and negative forces.
5. Identify four perspectives that affect strategic dynamics.

In this chapter, mapping the cardinal "who's who" of strategic planning and some of the necessary groundwork of strategic planning is discussed. Some of the more subjective and effective tools of the strategic planning process are reviewed, and potentially intimidating concepts, such as *force-field analysis*, are uncovered.

TOOL 1: STRATEGIC MAPS

Maps help you get from Point A to Point B using the most efficient route. They are universally understood and can be read and interpreted by people with a wide range of ages, learning styles, and cultural backgrounds. Likewise, strategic maps are easy to read and can be understood by people from several different departments and disciplines, and employees from differing learning styles and cultural backgrounds. Their purpose is to serve as a visual aid that clearly displays how their organization plans to get from where they are (Point A) to where they want to go (Point B).

These maps may be simple (a visual cut-to-the-chase of the major tenets) or complicated; they often show priorities and demonstrate how components of the plan are related and interrelated. Strategic maps can help people to picture one aspect of a project (such as a map that sets an algorithm for how to use an ECG), or they can be complex and include the overall picture (such as everyone and everything necessary to administer ECGs in a cardiac center that serves 50 clients per hour, 6 days per week). These maps help clarify direction, assist in planning, and display timelines and flow of responsibilities. Please see Figure 5-1 for a simple strategy map.

Simple maps may be used for general distribution, but more detailed strategic maps may be created for individual workgroups. For example, a hospital is planning an expansion. The general staff will need a strategic map that shows the overall project, departments affected, and timelines, and how the project will affect their work. The office of the chief executive officer (CEO) will have a detailed strategic map of the overall picture. (Please see Figure 5-2 for simple strategy map that may be used by the CEO, and Figure 5-3 for a more complex example of a strategic map based on the Balanced Scorecard of Kaplan & Norton, 1996.)

In this example, we have moved from a simple strategy map to one with more variables. Both are pretty straightforward and easy to follow. Let's take this a step further and look at a more detailed strategy map based on the Balanced Scorecard of Kaplan and Norton (please see Figure 5-3).

At first glance, this map is a little confusing and hard to follow. So let's study it. The map depicts a strategic financial theme for a healthcare organization. It

Figure 5-1   A simple strategic map demonstrating the components of a building project.

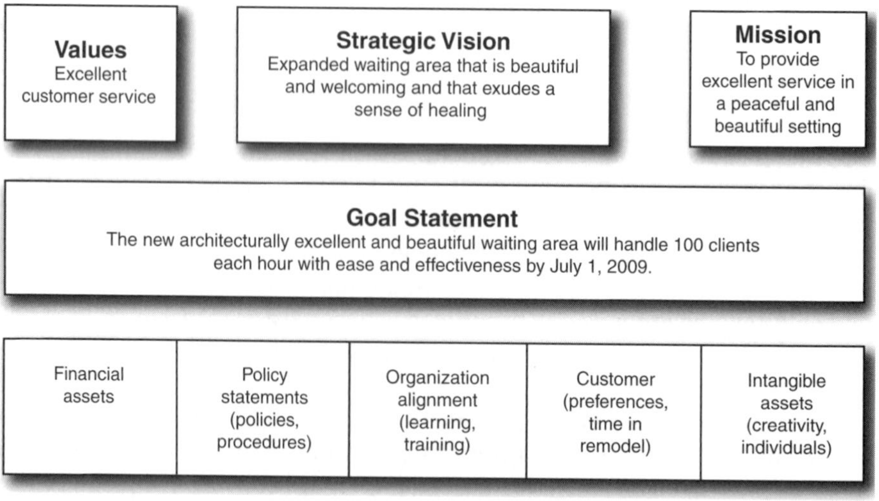

Values Excellent customer service	Strategic Vision Expanded waiting area that is beautiful and welcoming and that exudes a sense of healing	Mission To provide excellent service in a peaceful and beautiful setting

Goal Statement
The new architecturally excellent and beautiful waiting area will handle 100 clients each hour with ease and effectiveness by July 1, 2009.

Financial assets	Policy statements (policies, procedures)	Organization alignment (learning, training)	Customer (preferences, time in remodel)	Intangible assets (creativity, individuals)

Figure 5-2   Example of a strategic planning map: New building project.

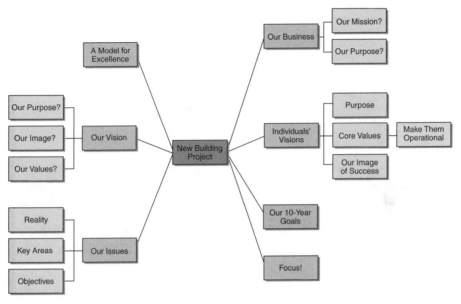

Source: Kaplan & Norton, 1996.

shows two main strategies: growth and productivity. These are related, but each has its own set of drivers. For example, both must show a return in capital; they have to make money. Both must be driven by the customer's needs and by indicators of quality. In order to *grow*, this company is planning to exceed the current market by 2–2.5% each year; they will use continual quality improvement measures and will increase capacity. To become more *productive*, they will look to employee development, continuous quality improvement (CQI), and customer satisfaction variables. At the foundation of each direction, the company will increase employees' awareness of the strategic plan by 50% as a means to create a motivated workforce. The arrows demonstrate how each piece to their plan is linked. Kaplan and Norton call this "balanced." As all aspects of the organization are linked.

Think about your checkbook. You may have a strategy to save $500 each month, but if you only look at your checkbook, you will not have a balanced view. What about any credit card debt or charges? Did you consider any automatic withdrawals? Have you planned for future spending (like the taxes that are due in 2 months)? Do you budget? How do you track being "on task," sometimes referred to as a "scorecard" (aligned with your strategy to save $500 each

Figure 5-3   A more detailed balanced scorecard strategy map of how a healthcare organization might conceptualize "balancing" (tying strategies, objectives, initiatives, and evaluation components into a whole as a means to link all aspects that affect an organization).

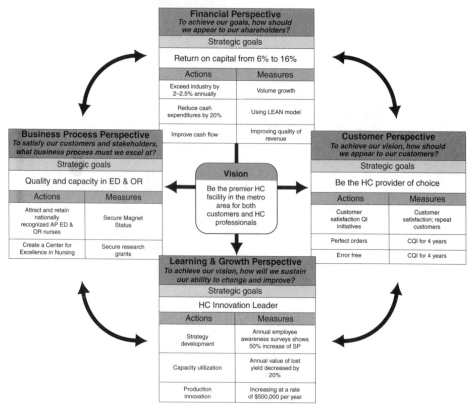

Source: Kaplan & Norton, 1996.

month)? A more complex integrated strategic map of your money plans will help you to understand the example of the strategies of this oil company (Figure 5-3). In our next section, we will look at how to use a strategic map, and we will use the saving of $500 each month as our objective.

How to Use a Strategic Map

Strategic maps are not unlike concept or mind maps; both show relationships between variables. Nurses are more familiar with concept or mind maps that show the relationships and logic in a thinking process. Nursing also employs flow charts; have you seen the old vital signs graphic sheets? Those showed the "flow" of a patient's condition in relation to his or her temperature, pulse, respirations, and blood pressure: a type of concept map. Strategic maps intend to show how aspects of a plan—the necessary resources, initiatives, and measures—are linked. These maps need to be clear and easy to follow, flow logically, and show how key resources are linked.

Strategic maps and concept maps may also be daunting if too many arrows and boxes clutter a page. We have all seen those concept maps gone amok. Does Figure 5-4 look familiar?

It really doesn't matter what the particular concept map in Figure 5-4 demonstrates because the reader gets lost trying to track all the connections. That isn't to say that some strategic planning maps do not become fairly convoluted out of necessity. But recognizing the fundamentals and purpose of a strategic map will help you to interpret, design, and participate in the mapping and the strategic planning process. Imagine a strategic map detailing how a medical-surgical unit will address quality improvement. Now imagine that strategic map looking like Figure 5-4. Staff would be left saying "Huh?" and buy-in and compliance would be a problem! When working with a strategic planning map, be sure to consider the intent and the audience.

Let's design our own strategic planning map using the $500-each-month savings example. Here, we would like you to practice using this strategy map to practice creating and participating in the mapping process. We have given you general headers, but you may design this as you see fit. We have assumed some values, a vision, and a mission. Please fill in the blanks in Figure 5-5 as a tool to learn strategy mapping.

> In Appendix 5a, we offer you a strategy map template that you can develop from your professional or personal values, vision, and mission. For more in-depth learning about strategic mapping, please read these books by Robert S. Kaplan and David R. Norton: *Strategy Maps*; *Alignment*; and *Translating Strategy into Action: The Balanced Scorecard*. Or, visit http://hbp.harvardbusiness.org/ep.

TOOL 2: STRATEGIC INTENT

Strategic intent is simply the alignment of what you want to accomplish and how it will be accomplished. Let's say that you want to save that $500, but you do not follow through. The intent may still exist, but the follow through, the

Figure 5-4   Concept map gone amok.

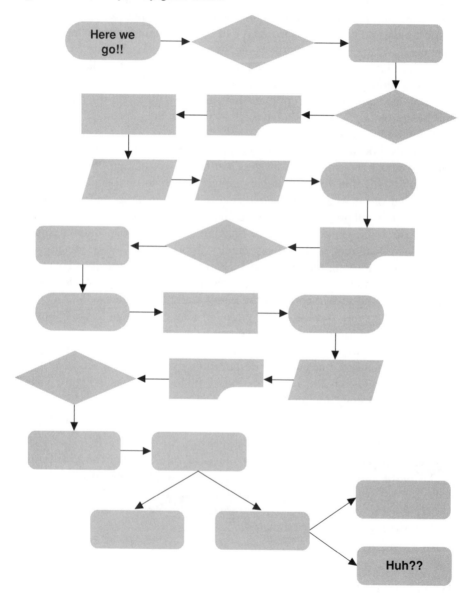

Figure 5-5   Create your own map.

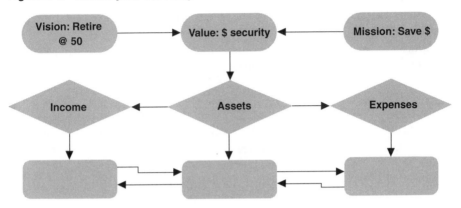

strategy, is omitted. Have you ever had a strategic intent to exercise, but some-where along the line, the intent was not partnered with the strategy, the imple-mentation? Perhaps you wanted to exercise to meet a cute guy at the gym, but when it turned out that the over-80 women monopolized the gym, your motiva-tion to exercise fell by the wayside. Strategic intent defines what is to be accomplished, but more important, it defines the purpose of the goal. Intent must be aligned with values. Imagine an administrator directing nursing to save $50 per patient by cutting back on the number of times a patient can use the bathroom; the intent is to save money, but the strategy is not strategic (leading toward the objective).

Strategic Intent: Align Purpose with Means

There are three paths to view strategic intent. First, there is the ethical view. The second is the view of "Do we have sufficient means to accomplish the pur-pose?" The third involves whether the organization works "in sync"—are the individual parts in alignment with the whole? Regarding the first view, the means does not justify the end; strategic plans are based first on values, a clear vision, and a mission that flows from these two underlying stated principles. This adage emphasizes the need to have all the means' (methods') ducks in a row based on the purpose.

In earlier chapters, we discussed potential contradictions between the values of care and those of business. Across our professional careers, we have been asked to jeopardize our purpose of care (as a means of saving money on staffing expenses), to work longer hours to cover shifts, or to work beyond our personal scope. You may have examples to add to this list. In this view of strategic intent, integrity is the issue.

> Consider your checkbook again. You want to save $500 each month, but it doesn't matter how you acquire that $500, so you just take it from your daughter's college savings account. The purpose and means are malaligned. The result must be reached without negating values.

The second approach to strategic alignment requires resource evaluation. Is there enough of everything, or is it realistically available, to accomplish the purpose? In the ideal scenario, you have all the necessary resources to realistically earn $500 extra each month even when considering all eventualities, current expenses, planned expenses, contingency plan needs, and external forces that may affect your money. In the less-than-excellent view of strategic intent, you are able to consider the same variables and, even though challenges are anticipated over the course of the project, the purpose will be accomplished. The process may not be seamless or easy, but with tight budgeting and by eating beans and rice, skipping lattes, and eliminating credit card debt, you will be able to save $500 each month: Strategic intent will be accomplished. In nursing, inadequate staffing levels are an obvious example of poor resource evaluation. Can you think of others?

The third type of alignment is that of everything working together in balance and heading in the same direction. The best analogy for this is a car whose tires and front end are in alignment: The car drives smoothly and uses fuel efficiently, the ride is comfortable, and passengers feel secure. A car that is out of alignment is wobbly, uses more fuel (inefficient), is uncomfortable for the driver and passengers, and lends to the feeling that the car will fall apart, which contributes to feelings of insecurity. Have you ever been in a work environment wherein management and resources were out of alignment? Tensions are usually high, egos are often engaged as a result of a lack of security, and the work "ride" is uncomfortable and wobbly! Before embarking on a change process, it is crucial to have buy-in—everyone driving in the same direction, and everyone with a safe vehicle that operates efficiently and smoothly.

Strategic intent encapsulating the concepts of alignment of ethics, alignment of resources, and alignment of purpose demands true leadership. Recall that management takes care of "things"; leadership takes care of setting direction and leading people. In a team approach, management will make sure that enough of everything exists, but leadership will assure that resources are engaged ethically and optimally on the right course. The strategic engineer is central to maintaining strategic intent in cooperation with management and leadership.

Unintended Consequences

Plan as thoroughly as we may—considering all forces, employing strategic thinking, imagining every eventuality—something still goes awry. In Chapter 4, we discussed developing contingency plans and disaster plans as a means of warding off unintended consequences. You get the flu shot, wash your hands, stay away from people who are infectious, and take good care of yourself, but you still get a flu bug. This is one type of unintended consequence—a force that couldn't be managed, even with best practices.

Another type of unintended consequence is associated with idiosyncrasies. Give aspirin (ASA) for a fever; instead, the child develops Reye's syndrome (of course, ASA is contraindicated in populations younger than 20). We know not to give children ASA, but how do we prepare for unintended consequences in a strategic process? Although the contingency and disaster plans may offer solutions, the truth is that unintended consequences often need to be dealt with as they arise: "Plan B." As nurses, we are quite adept at managing unintended consequences because we are, by nature, critical thinkers, and we deal in the business of hurdling obstacles. As you will see in a later section in this chapter ("Tool 4: Process Cycling"), when we come to a fork in the road, we will have to decide the best course by revisiting the strategic plan and deciding on the strategies that come out ahead of all others based on a continual assessment of values, vision, and mission.

TOOL 3: FORCE-FIELD ANALYSIS

No, this has nothing to do with *Star Wars*, but we think that the term sounds a little Darth Vader-ish!* Force-field analysis does have origins in the world of electromagnetism, wherein one body that is positive interacts with another that is negative. You have all experienced this with magnets; remember playing with magnets, and the ends of two magnets (poles) held next to each other

---

*Darth Vader is a fictional character in George Lucas's science fiction film saga *Star Wars*.

would attract or repel the other magnet? This is because of the electromagnetic field that they create, either positive or negative. Business has adapted the concepts of positive and negative magnetism and expanded the meaning to include positive forces that help (driving forces), and negative forces that hinder (restraining forces), the attainment of an enterprise's objectives.

Recall that driving forces come in many packages: internal drivers like EBP and research, knowledge, skills, management competence and leadership, available workforce, and the external forces of an organization (such as the economy, competitors and their advantage, technology, new diseases, and even emergency preparedness and terrorism). Restraining forces can be those very same things, but with a restraining effect. Forces, regardless of origin, have the potential to be positive or negative depending on their impact.

Emergency preparedness is a good example of a process that has been both a driving force and a restraining force. On the positive side, new funds and training have increased surge capacities, raised awareness, and increased competencies in mass causality management. On the negative (restraining) side, new workloads and training demands have stressed an already challenged healthcare workforce and added yet another layer to the equation of what a healthcare employee must demonstrate in order to be competitive. The art and science of emergency preparedness is ever evolving and is a moving target of competencies, making it difficult to establish the standard—the "bar"—that, once reached, signifies preparedness. Drivers and restraining forces in strategic planning are also not-so-easily quantified. We don't know what the process of emergency preparedness will require 5 years from now, but by thinking strategically, we may make an educated guess and think about how emergency preparedness will positively or negatively affect healthcare objectives in the future; we then "map" how these influences will be addressed.

Force-field analysis is the study of the positive and negative forces that affect an enterprise. It involves analyzing how those forces will play on that enterprise and against one another, and how they may change in the future. The analysis can be quite simple; for example, a force-field analysis of your checking account can reveal spending patterns that help (save $500 each month) and patterns that restrain (spend the extra $500 "just this one time"). Or, it can be quite complex and require a whole bevy of actuaries—for example, an anticipated merger of two large insurance companies.

Nurses already know how to conduct a type of force-field analysis; it is called the *nursing process*. Nurses continually make assessments, figure out what the assessments mean (diagnosis), determine outcomes or plans (objectives—what you want to happen), and implement and evaluate—all based on critical thinking. In the critical thinking process, nurses weigh all approaches and determine the best practices and most expedient methods, and they take

Recall that health care has an "extra" set of drivers in the myriad of reimbursement systems and the resulting regulations tied to the reimbursement schedules (most notably, Medicare and Medicaid). Health care is not an easy business; every business enterprise has challenges and unique competencies, but how many need full legal teams, infection control, sophisticated housekeeping, and state-of-the-art technology? How many deal with life-threatening issues minute by minute; require more training and education than any other industry; face threats of diseases and microbial resistance; must respond to multiple regulatory and accrediting agencies; and have to lead and manage a variety of disciplines and their unique needs, all under one roof? Although it all boils down to the point-of-care, there are many force fields acting on the patient, as well as on the clients and staff engaged in that patient's care.

measures to ensure the optimal client outcome—strategic thinking at its finest! By understanding the point-of-care needs, nurses are continually conducting a type of force-field analysis.

Nurses are at the point-of-care, but they have left the bigger picture of force-field analysis to others. As we all know, the point-of-care has become jeopardized because of restraining forces that have impacted health care and have filtered down to the bedside. Nurses are a cardinal part of the bigger picture of health care, and we must learn to engage in the process of force-field analysis or chance losing even more point-of-care (bedside) control. Remember the adage, "If we don't know where we are going, we'll probably end up somewhere else."

We'd like you to take a moment here and step back. Take a bird's-eye view of your healthcare employer:

- What do you see as the factors (drivers and restraining) that affect your job?
- Are they "all about you" (nursing), or are there other factors affecting your organization's ability to provide care?
- What is the local economy like?
- How is income generated, and who are the money-makers (usually a small elite group of specialty surgeons)?
- What other departments are making demands or expressing dissatisfaction?

Force-field analysis is an organized method of assessing all the players, the effect that those players have or may potentially have, and the strategies to best work with those players. Nursing, as with all components of health care, has both driving and restraining forces. Quality nursing care leads a healthcare organization in the direction of its objectives. Errors, employee dissatisfaction, workforce shortages, and poor retention rates all are restraining factors. Can you see that being a part of the force-field analysis has profound potential for strengthening nursing's role to empower the profession to be a part of the solution by challenging nursing to apply critical thinking (strategic thinking) inward to help solve the ills at the heart of care?

Let's tie strategy maps to force-field analysis. When looking at the previously mentioned example of a strategy map (Figure 5-3), do you see how the environment and safety are force fields that must be assessed and addressed in order to attain their goals (objectives) of growth and productivity? Strategy maps offer a visual of those variables that exert force on a project. Mapping cannot analyze those forces but does consider and demonstrate each force. Mapping helps all parties to see the larger picture by including all relevant forces (or drivers). Once project participants identify all the players and resources and then analyze how those players and resources act on, with, and against one another, the next phase of the strategic planning processes is to recognize that no process is static. The variables of today may change tomorrow. Identifying process cycling assessment tools is next.

TOOL 4: PROCESS CYCLING

Process cycling recognizes that change is the only constant. One simple example of process cycling is an academic year. Nursing faculty plan for academic year 2009–2010 given current knowledge and teaching (pedagogy) principles, but in November 2009, a new disease is discovered that holds the potential to cause a pandemic. Established content still has to be taught, pedagogy must adjust for new learning, and new evidence forces require that curriculum be adjusted.

> Another simple example of process cycling is to think about the example of your checkbook and consider the impact of the financial crisis of October 2008 on your financial situation. You probably reassessed your finances and came up with a Plan B based on new realities but in keeping with your original goals (objectives) to save $500 each month. The values, vision, and mission did not change; rather, new strategies were created to meet the new challenges.

Process cycling is just that: cycling of the process. The patient's temperature is 103°F; you develop strategies to decrease the patient's temperature, and 4 hours later, the temperature has spiked again. Begin again, and try to anticipate the cause and prevent complications. Very few processes are static; balance your checkbook on the first of the month, balance it the following month, and begin again with the next month's financial needs and realities: process cycling.

Process Cycling: Back to the Drawing Board!

Process cycling may be a normal, organic progression, like the checkbook example. Other process cycles carry threats and forces that may hinder the project and undermine the attainment of the goals or objectives. A dramatic example of a process cycle is the influenza (flu) season. The flu season comes between October and March every year. Some people will be vaccinated, but many will not receive the influenza vaccine. The vaccine may fail, and if so, healthcare workers may be the hardest hit. A new influenza strain may circumvent the globe within weeks. In 2007 H5N1, Avian Influenza, alarmed the world. The World Health Organization sharply increased the supply of pandemic influenza vaccine. The outbreaks of H5N1 set the world's public health workforce on high alert. Hospitals in India, Indonesia, Canada, and Hong Kong were put on isolation and quarantine. Strains of influenza continue to plague people across the United States every year. In 2009 H1N1, Swine Influenza, launched preparedness measures worldwide. The threat of a pandemic influenza is both ongoing and new as mutated influenza strains or strains that cross the animal-human barrier continue to evolve: process cycling.

Public health leaders and researchers studied and planned, looked for alternate care sites, determined the need for isolation and quarantine, communicated with all stakeholders, consulted with the public health experts worldwide, stayed in contact with airlines, highway, and railway systems personnel to track potentially infected travelers, and went back to the drawing board many times before the H5N1 and the H1N1 outbreaks were determined to no longer be a threat.

Your checkbook isn't as dramatic (we hope), but medical bills, household repairs, family emergencies, and a plethora of other forces come up, and you will go back to the drawing board time and time again to tweak your money plan. Process cycling is not a departure from the original values, vision, and mission; process cycling recognizes that life happens. As we plan, we do our best to consider every variable; we know that even though we paid this month's bills, they will show up again next month, and there may be unplanned expenses that we must consider over and over again.

Process cycling takes into account normal (organic) cycles, but it also considers those forces (drawn from the analysis of the force fields) that will influence a plan. It is not easy to show cycling on a strategy map with any detail; the map would become endless. One simple technique to demonstrate the force of cycling on a strategy map is with arrows. Please take a look at how Kaplan and Norton addressed cycling in Figure 5-3 with the use of arrows. Process cycling is reflected in the interrelatedness of growth and productivity; neither is static, and neither could be accomplished without the other. This is a nice segue into strategy dynamics, where we will look at defining and measuring the "pandemic forces" to minimize their impact on the strategic planning process.

TOOL 5: STRATEGY DYNAMICS

There are four perspectives (dynamics) that affect strategy dynamics: learning and growth, internal business processes, the customer, and money. This is a resource-based view of strategy. Strategy dynamics are "dynamic"—motive forces in action. Learning and growth are lifelong; business processes are continually undergoing quality assessment and are shifting from old top-down management systems to new, enlightened leadership systems. The customer is engaged in health care and is becoming increasingly better informed and responsible for his or her care. Money is influenced by reimbursement models, the Centers for Medicare and Medicaid Services, liability, national and local economies, population demographics, and the global market: dynamic.

The human resource is often the most dynamic variable in a strategic plan. Nursing's shift from being yesterday's labor workers to today's knowledge workers has necessitated the development of competency-based criteria in order to quantify the new professional parameters. Nursing used to be a set of easily measurable skills and skill sets. Find a nursing textbook from 1975, and you will see the emphasis on skills. Go to your local bookstore, and you will see that there are more "nursing procedure" books out there than almost any other type of nursing text (still addresses the labor worker). Things that are observable are easy to measure. Muscle-reflexor work is task oriented and has a circumscribed output: The suture is good and holds or it does not; a patient was bathed, IV competently inserted, and vital signs are stable, or not.

Assessment of knowledge, critical thinking, creativity, team processes, qualities of leadership, and other knowledge worker attributes has not been clearly defined and can be subjective. In considering strategy dynamics, learning and growth (human resource capability) are cardinal to a project's success. In today's healthcare marketplace, that learning and growth is not obvious. Nurses keep a pile of certificates and receipts from all the conferences, but do the pieces of paper assure learning and growth?

In her article, "The Dynamics of Strategy: Executive Summary" (2000), Kim Warren concluded that "capabilities . . . must make a difference" in how an organization grows and succeeds. The question is, how do we measure "learning" as valuable to improved outcomes and increased earnings in the strategic planning process dynamics? Stay tuned; the jury is still out, and workgroups across the world are trying to define competencies in the age of the information worker. Learning and growth are essential factors in the success of a change process, but as you may be well aware, many a manager questions the "value" of paying for courses, continuing education, advanced degrees, or release time for scholarly research or writing. Selling a banana for a 5% profit is measurable, but recovering the cost of knowledge is more elusive. Learning and growth are probably the most valuable components—dynamics—of any change process, but be prepared to offer quantifiable evidence as to the benefits: perhaps the most difficult to produce.

Internal business processes are those processes that an enterprise must excel at in order to satisfy both shareholders and the customers. In Chapter 2, we addressed the shift away from mission statements that focused on shareholder wealth but neglected to address customer satisfaction. The omission was corrected as healthcare businesses across the country came to the realization that without customer satisfaction, there was no shareholder wealth or sustainable shareholder wealth. Using strategic objectives (Chapter 4), new and existing business processes that will have an impact on both customer satisfaction and financial gain are identified.

Business processes are the "how things get done" within an enterprise. Policy and procedures for every department, legal considerations and forms, job and task descriptions and qualifications, accounting systems, management protocols and styles, purchasing and vendor relations, revenue streams, and even corporate culture are all examples of business processes.

Business is a process designed to make money; a product is sold that a consumer purchases. Business processes continually seek to measure effectiveness, consistency, and the timely delivery of the product in order to make a profit. Internal business processes (IBPs), a concept coined by Kaplan and Norton (1996) as a dynamic of the Balanced Scorecard (BSC), refers to the maximization of business processes as they impact the strategic planning process. Do more of what works and less of what doesn't, and identify new, better, and more ways to be more efficient, more consistent, and "on time."

The best examples of how businesses accomplish this are the IBPs designed by McDonald's. Hamburgers are cranked out across the world efficiently, consistently (a hamburger in Singapore looks and tastes just like a hamburger in Sioux Falls, South Dakota), and in a timely fashion (order your hamburger, drive to the pick-up window, and voila—a hamburger in packaging known worldwide). These IBPs are strategies that have directed the company's success. Healthcare administrators heed these lessons of "success"; diagnostic-related groups are an example of an IBP meant to increase profit and satisfy customers.

The other two dynamics of strategy dynamics are the customer and money. Satisfaction surveys, exit or discharge interviews, comment boxes, data collection on return visits, etc., all seek to assess customer satisfaction. Other familiar methods to assess customer satisfaction are outcome measures, incident/error reports, liability issues, hospital days, the occurrence of "never events," and profit and loss statements. Money is probably the most straightforward dynamic: revenues versus expenses, profits versus losses, assets versus liabilities. An enterprise needs more revenues, profits, and assets than expenses, losses, and liabilities. Having enough capital or knowing how to obtain sufficient capital in order to undertake a change process is fundamental to a project's success. Employees need to be paid, debts repaid, bills covered, and contingency plans funded.

Assessing strategy dynamics, making use of strategy maps, creating models that address process cycling, and employing other strategic planning tools such as force-field analysis can help to assure that pieces of the strategic plan are not overlooked. We have presented an overview of the principles of these tools. The best way to learn their use is to apply them to some of your everyday tasks. We have used the $500-per-month savings example for two reasons: (1) we can all relate to money, and (2) saving $500 per month is a bit of a stretch for most people and would require some serious strategic planning to implement.

Appendix 5a gives you an opportunity to try your hand at a strategy map. Appendix 5b is a template to help you identify process cycles and force-field analysis in nursing. Appendix 5c is a tool to help you apply the concepts of strategy dynamics. Take a moment to work with these forms before moving on to Chapter 6, where we will examine how to put strategic planning to work in nursing.

Perhaps one of the most recently used, but not yet widely understood, methods of healthcare improvement being employed by nurses is "lean health care," based on the famed Toyota Production System (TPS). The word *lean* may at first carry a negative connotation to nurses because it might imply the familiar and unpopular management tactics of cutting human and fiscal resources. Nothing could be farther from the truth! TPS/Lean is about cutting the unwanted "fat" (workarounds and reworking when what we need is not in place) and improving the "muscle" (the good thinking, experience, and compassion we bring to the job).

Borrowing the basic concept of reverence for the people who do the work and recognizing them as the local experts (who could possibly understand any work better than the people who do it?), TPS/Lean uses easy-to-learn, easy-to-teach methods of looking at processes of work with a new eye. Direct observation of the work in progress to identify *where the process doesn't support the work (and the nurse)* creates a fresh, objective, nonblaming approach to making improvements. Problems are always stated through the eyes of the patient, making the focus of improvement exactly where it should originate: from the patient experience. As a boundary tool for resolving process weaknesses that involve more than one department, the concepts and methods of TPS/Lean encourage documented and measured improvements that are patient focused and created in a collegial, nonthreatening environment. Because the improvements are done by the people doing the work, they carry with them ownership and accuracy. This is a perfect method for practicing shared governance.

Early research in the application of TPS/Lean to health care was done by a nurse, Cindy Jimmerson, with funding provided by the National Science Foundation through a grant to Montana State University's College of Engineering. The goals of the research included proving its efficacy in all departments of the healthcare organization, not just the brightest intensive care unit or the most efficient billing office. Results exceeded expectations, and over the 3 years (2001–2004) of the research period, interest in this program grew. The four major outcomes that Ms. Jimmerson recognized as accomplishments with the hundreds of improvement activities recorded were:

- Improved quality to the patient/decreased errors
- Decreased staff frustration related to process of work
- Reduced operating expenses
- Improved leadership skills

Since the conclusion of the research, Ms. Jimmerson has founded Lean Healthcare West, a group of healthcare professionals who practice and teach TPS/Lean in a very practical application. They have worked with more than 50 hospitals, clinics, physician office practices, and allied healthcare organizations to eliminate frustrating waste from work and improve delivery of health care to patients.

To learn more about the work of Lean Healthcare West, visit its Web site at http://www.leanhealthcarewest.com or call the Montana office at (406) 258-6535.

REVIEW QUESTIONS

1. What is the purpose of a strategic map?
2. What does the term *balanced* mean in strategic mapping?
3. Describe the three paths of strategic intention.

4. What is an unintended consequence?

5. Compare internal and external forces in force-field analysis.

6. What is process cycling?

7. What are the four perspectives that affect strategic dynamics?

REFERENCES

Kaplan, R., & Norton, D. (1996). *The Balanced Scorecard: Translating strategy into action.* Boston: Harvard Business School Press.

Warren, K. (2000). The dynamics of strategy: Executive summary. *Strategy Dynamics.* Retrieved November 9, 2008, from http://www.strategydynamics.com/products/Exec SummaryA4.pdf

Strategic Map Template

Template for designing your own strategy map:

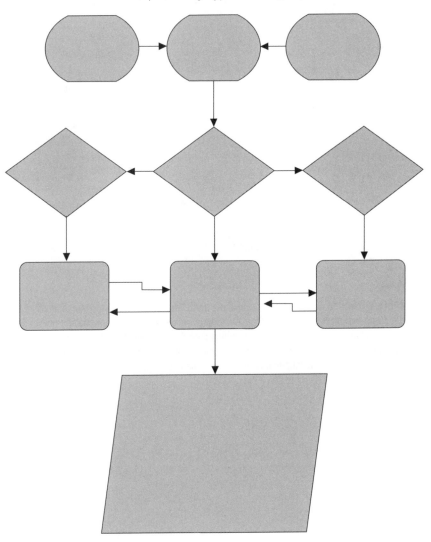

You may add or delete arrows and boxes. Remember, strategy maps show interrelatedness—"balance."

Identifying Process Cycles and Force-Field Analysis

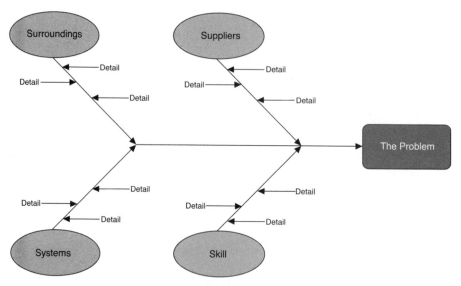

This is what is referred to as the 4 S's of Service diagram. The "details" are those forces (or force fields) that affect that particular service area. By adding arrows, you can demonstrate process cycling. For example, vendors need to deliver supplies continually. These suppliers can be central supply, pharmacy supply, or workforce supply. You get to decide which problem you will address, and that will dictate the skills, suppliers, surroundings (rooms, equipment, etc.), and systems (emergency medical records, policies, etc.) necessary to solve the problem.

Evaluation of Strategy Dynamics

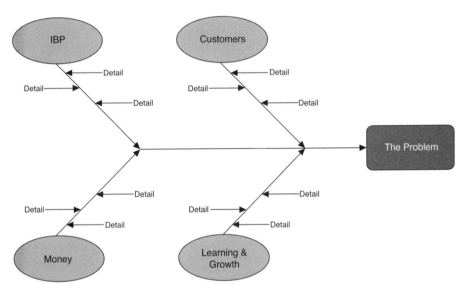

Identify a simple problem, like saving $500 each month, and think about what internal business processes (IBPs) you would need to change. What are the exact details affecting those IBPs? The customer would be you, but details about you would be helpful in determining the problem's solution. Do you balance your checkbook? Do you understand different savings options? What do you need to learn, or what areas of personal growth would be necessary to accomplish the goal? What money management practices would be necessary to solve the problem (i.e., the need to save $500 each month)? You can insert any problem and think of the details that will affect each of these dynamics.

CHAPTER 6

Strategic Planning: Why It's Not Just for the Boardroom Anymore

OBJECTIVES

1. Identify the value of the knowledge and industry work ethic.
2. Discuss methods of breaking down the stereotypic prejudices nursing has created, illuminating the us-versus-them mentality.
3. Recognize nurses as stakeholders.
4. Describe the shift of industrial-age management to knowledge-age management.
5. Review metaleadership.
6. Evaluate the quality and intent of job descriptions and the policy and procedure content.
7. Discuss the impact of nursing culture as a locus of control.

Nursing has been intent on addressing the plethora of internal issues necessary to bring nursing into maturity and to ensure quality care. Along a parallel path, one that controls nursing in many areas, the world of healthcare business was also maturing—an entity process that became distinctly separate. Health care transitioned from a model based on charity to a model based on Wall Street. A chasm between care and administration developed, creating lines of contention and misunderstanding. The change was so dramatic, quick, and powerful that it left nursing on the periphery of decision-making. This chapter offers a global view of the competencies necessary to bridge the chasm.

WELCOME TO THE KNOWLEDGE AGE!

Do you consider yourself a knowledge worker or an industry worker? Or a little of both? If you asked your peers, your manager, and your administrator that question, what do you suppose the answer would be? Which do you think the members of the board consider themselves to be? What about administrators, accountants, and quality control specialists? Has someone you work with ever referred to you as a "worker bee"? Have you used that term to refer to yourself?

Recalling that the average age for a nurse is hovering around the mid to late 40s, we know that many of you grew up in the age of "hard work never hurt anyone." Physical labor was, and is, considered somehow "more" American. "Work ethic" was, and is, associated with hard physical occupations in which the industry worker was/is a national hero while the management was/is demonized. This has created a type of a "working class" credo of martyrdom borne out of the trials and hardships of the industrial revolution and age. These trials and hardships are not really relevant to today's nursing habitat, but we have clung to the us (worker) versus them (administration) culture nonetheless. We strongly encourage a robust work ethic. One pervasive concern in today's workforce is the seeming lack of work skills—a type of entitlement among some people that work "owes" them something. We resolutely embrace positive work practices and ethics; we just don't want self-limiting beliefs to keep your sphere of influence small.

Continuing to identify predominantly with the industrial era in many ways, Michele is a rancher and values hard (physical) work, and she understands the "blue collar" values of her community. For years, her identity as a nurse flowed from her ability to be the "hardest, most dependable" (etc.) worker. LeAnn has a family heritage in forest products and also is able to identify with being an industry worker (as opposed to a knowledge worker). Personally and professionally, our identities have shifted to knowledge workers. We value both; one is not better than or more important than the other.

The levels and degrees that populate the nursing profession offer labels of membership into these fictitious categories (we're not condoning this; this is just an observation over many years): LPN and ADN = blue collar; BSN, MSN, AP, etc. = white collar. Creating this us and them within the profession has had deleterious effects—a type of "nurseism," a prejudice among nurses, that has eroded nursing's credibility in many sectors. For example, Michele recently worked with a senator's aide who said, "Why ask nursing, they can't even get along within the profession . . . it seems like every nursing group you talk to has their own opinions." We think that this terrible news flows in part from the internal cultural disconnects: our own "us versus them," self-inflicted nurseism.

Crossing the chasm between the two worldviews is not a seamless process; both have their own cultural paradigms—characteristics, belief systems, and language. Nursing has historically aligned itself with the blue-collar worker and considered management as the white-collar worker, and ne'er the two shall meet. Blue-collar workers bowl, and white-collar workers play golf. Yes, this is a silly stereotype, but what we want you to think about is your identity as a nurse. We believe that white-collar workers bowl and blue-collar workers play golf, and who cares? But if, as a nurse, you have aligned yourself—boxed yourself in—with either view, we want you to stop doing that.

We are seeing a changing of the nursing workforce guard as new nurses who identify with white-collar knowledge workers mingle with older (seasoned) nurses who culturally identify with blue-collar industry workers. This phenomenon has created some of nursing's internal conflicts. Those who view themselves solely as knowledge workers may have the tendency to place themselves "above" physical labor and spend disproportionate work time theorizing and neglecting necessary physical skills and tasks. Those who view themselves solely as industry workers may tend to pride themselves on work ethic and excellent task completion but not be current in principles of contemporary nursing practice. Obviously, a competent and contemporary nurse identifies with both worldviews.

We need to remember that nurses (you) are not labels, degrees, and levels; they (you) are providers of care. We would also like you to know that "us" and "them" are obsolete, fictitious categories. As a provider of care, you are entitled to participate in decision-making processes, and you have the right and responsibility to sit at the boardroom table where you can offer powerfully articulate advocacy for care. If you are a nurse at any level (LPN, ADN, BSN, MSN, PhD), you are a knowledge worker. You are also an industry worker, but above all, you are a provider of care. Please do not disallow yourself full participation in decision-making processes as a result of a fictitious label. The American Nurses Association (ANA) defines one of the essential features of professional nursing as "influence on social and public policy to promote social justice." The ANA's definition of professional nursing includes "advocacy in the care of individuals, families, communities and populations" (ANA, 2003). Learn the necessary skills of business processes and let your voice be heard! Welcome to the knowledge age!

OPENING THE PROCESS TO ALL STAKEHOLDERS

There are people who function optimally when given clear guidance, and they prefer to be task oriented; they are not interested in or comfortable with team and decision-making processes. You know who you are; be true to that, but be sure that your abilities and position are not externally defined. Each person has unique abilities, styles, cultural beliefs, and expertise. There is a place for every ethical, legal, and moral style of care within the professional home of nursing. As a nurse, you are a stakeholder. Where you personally and professionally fit within the arena of health care is part of your own strategic plan, which should be intelligently and compassionately guided by career advisors (those you know and trust within your enterprise). Remember to use the optimal resource (a.k.a. the "human" resource).

Nursing schools are generic and tend to produce "nurse units"—a skill and knowledge set that can successfully pass the state board exams. All schools of nursing have a medical-surgical orientation (ultimately, we teach to the test, because NCLEX pass rates are a determining factor in accreditation). Many nurses continue to identify with competencies ("I am good at IV" or "I'm the code nurse"). Nurses are more than skills and bring a kaleidoscope of powerful attributes to the table. Discovering a voice for those abilities and strengths that are uniquely yours is an opportunity for every nurse in this new century.

The term *stakeholders* is often used to refer to board members and shareholders but now includes everyone engaged in and affected by care. In the past two decades, the term *stakeholders* in health care has expanded to include the patient (client, consumer, resident), the community, payers, regulatory and advisory bodies, and workers. As a nurse, you are a stakeholder; as the largest healthcare workforce, you are an essential, indispensable primary stakeholder.

THE INFORMATION CASCADE SHOULD FLOW UP AND DOWN: CHANGED MANAGEMENT PARADIGMS OF THE "KNOWLEDGE AGE"

The shift from industrial-age management practices and micromanagement to management based on quality leadership is the work revolution of the 21st century. Indeed, "Management" has become a new discipline and field of study as it transitions from a focus on inventory, faculty control, budget manipulation, and production quotas to a focus on quality and leadership of the knowledge worker. The information age of steel and plastic "things" is easily measured, but the value and capacity of knowledge requires new business practices. A poignant example of this phenomenon is the billions of dollars made off of virtual reality; it is impossible to measure the value and capacity of the Internet. Health care is a part of this immeasurable new reality.

Parallel to changes in the way business is being conducted philosophically and intellectually is the rise of new models of business practice—models that focus on leadership instead of management. Some of the most successful examples of such business models have come out of Japan. Two examples are Hoshin Kanri (or compass [specific direction] control) and the Toyota Model (14 principles that drive quality improvement and increase production and capacity). Both models seek to improve strategic direction and processes, but they do so in a manner divergent from the old industrial model; both pursue employee engagement and principles of empowerment.[1]

Another shift in how business is being conducted involves the paradigm of metaleadership: *Meta* refers to "underlying meaning." Nurses are familiar with metacommunication, or the message-within-the-message form of communication. Metaleadership expands on this idea, taking leadership to an integrated process that includes all stakeholders and wherein disciplines work together, as opposed to working in "silos" (i.e., doing their own thing). Health care once employed the model of interdisciplinary staffing; all relevant parties got together to discuss and review challenges in client care and to problem-solve. Somewhere along the way, this collaborative effort faded away, and many healthcare professionals began working in silos, isolated in practice from other specialty silos. As metaleadership once again gains momentum, nurses (key stakeholders) will be engaged in the decision-making processes, and each nurse will need to be prepared to function as a competent member of a business team.

These principles, or some similar leadership strategies, are the tools that administrators are being taught and are discussing. The new leadership styles are 21st-century drivers of the way care is delivered. Nurses would be well advised to make themselves familiar with these shifts and keep a hand on the pulse of changes in business. As a nurse, you are a stakeholder; make it your business to know your business!

In the industrial-age models, direction and decisions flowed "down." Healthcare business frameworks relied on a top-down flow of information. In this age of information, with more and more workers engaged in knowledge pursuits, the information is beginning to flow "up" through the ranks. Where once autocratic management "told" healthcare workers how to provide care, now educated workers provide collaborative direction in how care is delivered. This is the beginning of dialogue that flows down and up. Business-based administration does not have all the answers to the multiple challenges in care. Enlightened managers and leaders increasingly are looking to the healthcare workforce to help design solutions. Be sure that you are ready. If asked today, what would you voice as solutions to the "nursing crisis"?

If administrators and schools of management are shifting their competencies by embarking on a new learning curve, then the workforce needs to hop on that same curve. Nursing got sorely left behind in the national shifts that

---

[1]To learn more about Hoshin Kanri, please visit http://www.mcts.com/Hoshin-Kanri.htm; to learn more about the Toyota Model, please visit http://wcco.com/specialreports/Methodist.Hospital.lean.2.352128.html or pick up a copy of *The Toyota Way: 14 Management Principles from the World's Greatest Manufacturer* (2004), by Jeffrey Liker.

flowed from the Balanced Budget Act; let us not be left out again. The world of business is changing all around us nationally and globally; be a part of that change, or become obsolete and ineffectual. What is one strategy that you would implement to improve care in your facility? How will you communicate that "up"?

CASCADING UP: CREATING THE FLOW

> *"Be the change you wish to see in the world."*
> —Mahatma Gandhi, 1869–1948

So, a nurse is both a knowledge worker and industry worker, with a shift toward more fully participating in the information age; nurses are key stakeholders; new business models both allow and encourage dialogue that flows down and up; and nurses are more than their NCLEX exam: Nurses are individuals with diverse capabilities and unique ways of being. The 21st century offers new opportunities and challenges to give voice to and express care like never before. The cement boundaries of care are crumbling, and nurses are poised to respond to this new era. Fifteen million nurses is a pretty big group—the largest healthcare workforce.

If nursing ever truly realizes and seizes this capacity, the potential for positive change will be unsurpassed by any other organized effort. Start creating that communication flow up by employing sound principles of business through clarifying values, creating a vision, identifying a mission, and setting strategic objectives aligned with your organization—or create your own. You are a knowledge worker in the information age. You are a key stakeholder in health care. You are capable of learning anything in order to accomplish your purpose of care; be the change.

PROCESS MANAGEMENT AND LEADERSHIP DECISION: THE NURSE'S SPHERE OF INFLUENCE AND LOCUS OF CONTROL

Process management, as defined in Chapter 5, refers to how things work. In relation to strategic planning, these business processes are specifically those that will help an enterprise to excel within the marketplace.

Can you identify processes within your organization or school that have been implemented to improve outcomes or address quality problems?

In health care these process controls are often found in the policy and procedure (P&P) manuals that get dusted off or reviewed periodically (especially during audits or surveys). These P&P manuals are the holy grails of procedures; scope of practice, grievance processes, how to access the Internet, and any number of processes that need standardization across disciplines—such as hand-washing—get corralled in these extensive documents. Between the covers of these binders or Internet files (as the case may be in this technology age) lies a powerful locus of control defining nursing. Nursing gets boiled down to one- or two-page descriptions of care and all the peripheral practices that surround care.

Some enterprises gather their P&P from generic computer databases or software programs and place their institution's heading on the documents. Have you ever thought about the impact that P&Ps have on nursing? They define you; they are a locus of control tool in process management.

Who establishes your facility's P&P? This set of documents is a part of the strategic plan for your facility, or should be. These documents offer guidelines, direction, and parameters (scope) for care practice. Are they complete? Do your institution's P&Ps cover everything that a nurse is in the information age, or is the P&P manual holding nursing in the industrial age? At the end of the day, those manuals are binding. Their purpose is to maintain quality and standardize practice, but do they prescribe nurses as knowledge workers or as industry workers? This essential component of process management may be holding nursing back. Take a look at your facility's or unit's P&P manual and make a list of how many entries require a knowledge worker and how many compartmentalize nursing as an industry worker profession.

Job descriptions themselves offer another locus of control. What does yours say about you? Can you recall? (Did you even really read it?) When was the last time the job descriptions were reviewed, and by whom? Some descriptions are generic, some are micromanagement devices, and some are filled with legalese. Still others are representative of a knowledge-based worker in the 21st century. Although nursing unions have often reclaimed this vital locus of control, most nurses are handed job descriptions, often created by non-nurses. Which is yours? Have you ever negotiated your job description? If the last time that you saw your job description was at your evaluation, ask for a copy (if you don't already have one) and interpret its intentions.

WHAT DOES YOUR JOB DESCRIPTION SAY ABOUT YOU AND WHAT YOU DO AS A NURSE?

An obvious process locus of control resides in the management and leadership systems of your facility. Who is in charge of what, and how? What are the consequences of their actions? We all have seen a flow chart depicting the CEO, various "vice" positions, on to middle management, on down to charge nursing, and finally to staff positions. Most healthcare enterprises continue to rely on hierarchies as their system framework. The military relies on hierarchies; theirs indeed is a very rigid chain of command. Some managers tout open-door management. Teams are becoming very popular. Unit management, integrated leadership, shared governance, centralized management, and pod systems management are some frameworks you may have worked with, or your facility may have designed and labeled its own unique process management tools to create locus of control (defined in the P&P!).

At the unit level, many system frameworks have been tested. In the late 1970s and early 1980s, a movement toward "primary care" meant that only RNs would staff a floor and do all cares. There were no certified nursing assistants (CNAs), healthcare assistants (HCAs) or personal care attendants (PCAs) in this primary care model. Nurses designed the notion that they would provide care in every form, from bed baths to central venous pressures. It did not take long for dissatisfaction and exhaustion to set in, and the system was abandoned. Nursing has tried other versions of primary care— for example, when a national declaration was made that only BSNs were nurses. This too has not been sustainable because of a lack of program opportunities and the needs of the students pursuing a career in nursing. As discussed in Chapter 2, reimbursement models have defined value of practice. When the dialogue of "entry into practice" became about BSN preparation, nonhospital enterprises, and recognition of the demographics of the nursing profession (Who are the students? Where do they come from? What are their backgrounds?) were left out of the equation. Articulation, or career laddering, models have never been fully actualized within the vocation-profession of nursing.

A fourth locus of control is the healthcare culture itself. Nursing has its own unique culture. In the not-too-distant past many nurses smoked, were overweight, starched everything, held a gauntlet over students' and new nurses' necks, and stood when a physician entered a ward (we all should be aghast and embarrassed that a few of our fellow nursing students were becoming nurses in order to marry doctors—bizarre!), and nurses never discussed anything related to financial matters. Nursing culture is a characterization of the prevailing culture. Think about the differences in ways of being and beliefs between nursing units. Can you illuminate cultural practices and beliefs that are unique to ICU nursing, long-term care nursing, office nursing, and public health nursing? How are you "controlled" by that culture? Review Table 6-1 and think about the way that culture both negatively and positively impacts (locus of control) your practice.

Table 6-1   Cultures Within Nursing

Unit	Belief	Practice	Knowledge	Customs
Critical Care	Superior nursing	Continual learning of technology	Specialty in assessment modalities	Isolated from other units; share stories of dramatic rescues, cool stethoscopes
Pediatrics	Love children; specialized knowledge and ability	Ability to "marry" skilled nursing with therapeutic "mothering"	Specialty in age-appropriate interventions & assessment	Cute uniforms, teddy bears on stethoscopes, systems to weather child traumas
Clinic Nursing	Family centered, support the medical model	Prevention, early treatment, education	Specialty in generalist practice	Office relationships, pride in efficient process systems
Public Health Nursing	Community-based empowerment of wellness	Prevention, early treatment, education, high-level wellness	Health promotion and disease prevention specialists	Navy blue, war stories of monumental hygiene disasters, great STD stories
Long-Term Care	Value of elders, end-of-life, and dignity; overworked and undervalued	Gerontology-specific competencies and tremendous time management with excessive caseloads	Gerontology-specific competencies and assessments	Custom of not engaging or collaborating with other nursing specialties, few cool nursing toys or identity

In addition to a prevailing culture based on practice area, there is also a "style" culture that acts as a locus of process control. Take a moment to identify the general culture that dominates your work environment. At one university where Michele worked, there was a cultural expectation that faculty would work 10 hours each day and still have grading and lecture preparation at home. Weekend, holiday, and summer work was also expected (without pay, of course). It is fascinating how many nurses are martyrs; we don't say, "No thank you." Can it be that the culture of nursing is a little codependent and populated with rescuers? We'll save that can of worms for another book, but please consider how that cultural way of being has either helped or hindered nursing's professional progression and ability to participate in business processes. This pervasive locus of control influences the future directions in nursing.

These external loci of control are easily quantifiable and definable. Although the most important locus of control is not quantifiable, it is definable: your internal locus of control. This atlas of your personal and professional culture is your internal worldview—your beliefs, practices, knowledge, and customs. These are the property of the knowledge worker and cannot be owned by anyone else (although management is trying to corral "knowledge" by defining competencies). In the industrial age, factory workers were hired based on measurable physical attributes; there weren't many frail miners or auto workers. Do your physical attributes and psychomotor abilities define you? Here is an exercise to help you actualize this important reality:

Write a job description for Stephen Hawking:

_____

_____

Write a job description for Florence Nightingale during the years of her confinement late in her nursing career:

_____

_____

STRONGER THAN BEFORE, A STRENGTHENING MOMENTUM

Knowledge worker, industry worker, stakeholder, empowered communicator, process manager, cultural revolutionary, and an individual driven by a formidable internal locus of control—nurses are ready to claim their place as a business partner. Nursing is stronger than before and is gaining momentum in the pursuit of professional excellence. Some nurseism roadblocks are standing in our way. Think deeply about the tenets of this short chapter; hold your limiting beliefs up to the light, examine them from every angle, determine your own truth about possibility, and critically think about the current truths in nursing. Do these beliefs still serve you or the profession well? Even if you see nursing as a blue-collar workforce with no voice, we challenge you to overturn that paradigm as we move to the next chapters and the details of the strategic planning process.

REVIEW QUESTIONS

1. How is the profession of nursing both an industrial-age and knowledge-age profession?
2. What is metaleadership?
3. Knowledge-age management has been charged with managing what?
4. How do policies and procedures define nursing?
5. What is meant by information flow "down" and "up"?
6. How does nursing culture act as a locus of control in the nursing profession?

REFERENCES

American Nurses Association (ANA). (2003). *Nursing's social policy statement* (2nd ed.). Silver Spring, MD: Nursebooks.org.

Liker, J. (2004). *The Toyota Way: 14 management principles from the world's greatest manufacturer.* New York: McGraw-Hill.

CHAPTER 7

The Three Key Elements of the Strategic Planning Process: A Vision That Guides Nursing's Future Action

──────── OBJECTIVES ────────

1. Identify the three main components of a strategic review.
2. Compare strategic review to the nursing process.
3. Review the impact of positive and negative forces in a strategic review.
4. Discuss the eight steps of the strategic review process.
5. Evaluate visions for nursing from a variety of professional organizations.
6. Identify tools for obtainable goals that relate to the desired vision and values.
7. Distinguish the roles needed to create and implement a strategic plan.

This chapter takes the previously discussed conundrums and applies strategic planning processes to the needs of nursing. The reader will follow a case study for each element, identifying the key roles, and have the opportunity to apply that element to his or her unique scenario and expertise.

ELEMENT 1—THE STRATEGIC REVIEW: WHERE IS NURSING NOW?

> *"Born to see, meant to look"*
> —Faust, 1831

The Strategic Review Process

In Chapter 4, we discussed the strategic review (also referred to as the "environmental assessment" or "situational analysis") as a potentially sensitive procedure that reveals the tender underbelly of processes and people. The first three chapters are a strategic review of where nursing is now. Although we have spoken frankly about nursing, please realize that we are talking about ourselves as "every nurse." We are emotionally, intellectually, financially, and spiritually invested in nursing; there is no "us" and "them" in this process. As we discover the beneficial applications of the business process, please engage in dispassionate reasoning. If the examples we share do not resonate with you, pull one from your professional experience to apply these principles.

A strategic review (SR) often looks at past, current, and future performances, as well as opportunities, outside forces, and internal forces. Trends and issues have been the driving force of this text. Take a moment now to think about your past professional performance, how you feel your performance is today, where opportunities for improvements exist, and what you want to accomplish. What external factors affect your performance? Think about your optimal professional performance. What are your internal barriers to achieving your desired level of performance? Congratulations, you just conducted a strategic review!

The SR is not a haphazard set of opinions, nor is the process based on feelings; however, there are both subjective and objective components. The process is a methodically pragmatic look at factors that determine market position, performance, and competitive edge. To translate into nursing parlance, it is the assessment phase of the nursing process (NP), which is "an evaluation or an appraisal of a condition . . . and the process of making that evaluation" (*Mosby's*, 2005). The process encompasses the art of focused assessment, knowing *what* to assess and having the ability to interpret the findings.

In the SR process, team members systematically identify specific elements, determine which characteristics of those elements are pivotal to assess, and then use or access (such as contracting an accountant) knowledge to interpret the discovered information. The SR process is familiar to anyone who files a tax return. No matter how hard a person may try to cloak his or her financial picture, the Internal Revenue Service tax reporting system requires an investigation (looking), compilation (knowing what to look at), and interpretation of income (knowledge and skills to understand findings). Most people manage to corral the "looking at" and the "knowing what to look at," and some brave souls prepare their own taxes, but many of us need to access a tax accountant to interpret the findings properly.

An SR may take minutes or months, depending on the extent and scope of the strategic process intent. Regardless of the breadth of a project, some simple steps and principles are required. Just as you would not assess vital signs but omit lung sounds on a patient complaining of shortness of breath, skipping parts of the SR will likewise render incomplete or inaccurate data, leading to faulty conclusions. Let's look at the principles and steps of the SR process.

The SR process encompasses three main components: structures, processes, and governance. *Structures* refers to how an enterprise is organized. *Processes* refers to how discipline-specific actions occur (recall the P&P manuals). *Governance* refers to how decisions are made based on organizational rules and authority. See Table 7-1.

The scope of the review must be defined when strategic planning is conceived. The purpose of the plan drives the scope of the review. For example, is the review meant to look at the big picture, or a specific structure, process, or governance? Or is it meant to be a completely new design? In the eight steps in Table 7-2, we used the example of an epidemiological dilemma that was very narrow in scope; day-to-day processes were reviewed (structure and governance were not measured). If pseudomonas-related deaths occur across units, including inpatient and outpatient areas, both systems and process will need to be reviewed. Structures, processes, and governance need to be reviewed if the planning process goal is to improve the infection rates throughout an organization.

Reviews are truth seeking; however, before any questions are asked, the enterprise needs to ask itself, "Are we healthy enough to do this?" In Chapter 4, we looked at a "quick check" to determine readiness to undertake strategic planning. If the enterprise is in crisis, some business authorities suggest that strategic plans be forgone. In Chapter 1, we discussed the many faces of the nursing crisis. Because nursing is broken, should we wait for a professionally healthier time to envision a better future? We'll let you answer that for yourself. Only you can decide if, how, and when you will engage in a cathartic

---

Table 7-1   The Three Principles of the Strategic Review Process

1. SR is not static, done once and never thought about again. SR is an ongoing process of continual improvement. Example: Assessing MRSA rates and contributing factors in an ICU once each year will not reveal etiology and incidence, nor will outcomes improve; infection control is a continual quality improvement process.
2. The SR is meant as a tool to test, learn about, and revamp strategies—what is working, what isn't, and what is being overlooked.
3. The SR is "appropriately encompassing." Human nature gives attention to those things that make us look good and neglects or minimizes those things that make us look bad. Remember, this is a reality-seeking process, not a "this is how we want it to look" process.

Table 7-2   The Eight Steps to the Strategic Review Process

1. Identify the purpose of the strategic planning process; what is/are the objective(s) to be accomplished? Example: decrease in errors, improved retention, increased income, greater market share.
2. Identify strategic review (SR) team members or active "lookers"; achieve the appropriate skill and knowledge mix and include members who are vested in the process being reviewed. Example: An intensive care unit (ICU) nurse and a long-term care (LTC) nurse should be on a team that seeks to improve outcomes and decrease cost associated with nosocomial-related illness in persons admitted to LTC posthospitalization in an ICU.
3. Identify what will be assessed (looked at); again, assessment must be thorough in order to be pertinent. Example: Looking at Methicillin Resistant Staphylococcus Aureus (MRSA) rates singularly in relation to LTC disregards the shared responsibility for clients across facilities, especially given the astonishingly high MRSA rates in ICUs.
4. Identify, develop, or access expertise to interpret what is discovered. Example: It wasn't until 2000 that epidemiologists from the Centers for Disease Control and Prevention's (CDC's) hospital infection control division were able to determine that nurses with long fingernails had inadvertently transmitted bacteria to infants in a neonatal intensive care unit (NICU) at The Children's Hospital in Oklahoma City; as a result, eight infants died between 1997 and 1998 (Altman, 2000).
5. Interpret findings. Example: *Pseudomonas aeruginosa* was either transmitted to or from the susceptible babies. It was then spread in this high-risk population by the nurses who had long fingernails, which harbored the genetic type of pseudomonas that killed the infants.
6. Make recommendations. Example: The team investigating the infant deaths recommended against the use of artificial and long fingernails in intensive care and transplant units (Moolenaar et al., 2000).
7. Set strategies. Example: Although there were other variables in this investigation, the only link was nurses with long or artificial nails; the hospital administration strategy now restricts the use of artificial and/or long nails; CDC guidelines now state that operating room personnel should not wear long nails and concluded that short natural fingernails in all healthcare workers may decrease the incidence of hospital-acquired infections (Moolenaar et al., 2000).
8. Assess strategy success. Example: No deaths from the pseudomonas have been reported in The Children's Hospital in Oklahoma City since requiring the nurses in the NICU to have short natural nails—a successful strategy.

innovation in care and whether that change is to a structure, a process, or governance.

Strategic reviews ask questions. Better questions are followed by better answers. The first question is, Are we committed to change? The second question is, What is our purpose (based on values)? And the third question is, What is our vision? These three questions are at the heart of every stage of the strategic planning process; remember that a journey of a thousand miles begins with a single step—as long as you step in the right direction.

Table 7-3 is an example of questions that may be asked in an SR. The questions vary depending on the scope and intent of the strategic plan.

As discussed in Chapter 4, one tool that is commonly used in SR is the SWOT process: Identify strengths, weaknesses, opportunities, and threats. Figure 7-1 offers a SWOT template that you can use. A SWOT analysis identifies forces that affect the SR process. Part of SR is called a force-field analysis. Figure 7-2 offers a visual of the SR process using force-field analyses.

Strategic reviews are usually conducted by management as a precursor to the strategic planning process. This process must be thorough, lest faulty information misdirect. Imagine using only one lead of an EKG machine in the cardiac care unit to record the hourly rhythm interpretations; such faulty information would endanger clients. Now imagine that only 1 out of every 4 nurses knows how to conduct a physical assessment. *No* nurse left behind. It takes

---

Table 7-3   Example of Questions Asked in a Strategic Review

- What is the purpose of the review? What do we hope to learn?
- Is this a problem-based plan (such as a quality improvement initiative) or a plan intended to redesign structures, process, and/or governance?
- What are the product/products that we seek to improve?
- Is there financial viability?
- What responsibilities and decision-making authority do involved persons and programs have?
- What are the strategic team members' rights, responsibilities, and roles?
- How will performance be measured?
- Are structures aligned with purpose?
- Are processes aligned with purpose?
- How is communication managed within the enterprise and externally?
- What are corporate- and discipline-specific cultural considerations? (We all know that nurses have their own "culture.")
- Empirical data are "easy" to analyze; how will affective and subjective information be evaluated?
- Who needs to be included (individuals, departments, consultants, management, etc.)?
- Strengths?
- Weaknesses?
- Threats?
- Opportunities?

Figure 7-1   SWOT template.

	Internal	External
Positive	Strengths	Opportunities
Negative	Weaknesses	Threats

a village to achieve strategic alignment from top to bottom. The SR may begin with "management," but nurses must have a seat at the management table. Directions in care must be set by the care experts, whom we know must include nurses.

In the SR, it is crucial to have the right people asking the right questions. Have you ever had a report come from the "top" on how you are doing? Was it accurate? Did it appropriately reflect your work, strengths, and weaknesses? Did the report, perhaps in the form of an evaluation, represent your areas of opportunity for growth, and outside forces impeding your growth? The SR team must comprise people who can best answer the questions. Just as you are the best judge of your strengths, weaknesses, opportunities, and threats in your professional life, so it is that nurses are the best judges of how to ask the key questions in an SR of care. Nurses need to make the "assessment."

A universally fundamental knowledge and skill set in nursing is assessment. Nurses are trained to look and interpret what they see. Without honed assessment skills and knowledge, nurses would be useless. The nurse's value is his or her ability to assess, interpret, and respond to the infinite scenarios surrounding care. The SR of care turns those eyes inward on nursing itself. So let's do it: Here is the SR process, using nursing as the subject to be assessed.

Figure 7-2   Strategic review employing a force-field analysis template.

Each force is scored according to its "magnitude," ranging from 1 (*weak*) to 5 (*strong*).

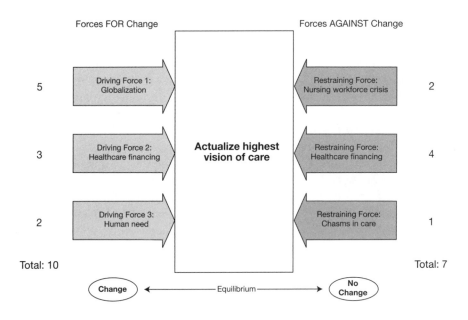

Note: We created sample numbers for the scoring; you can set your own values for importance.

ELEMENT 2—CLARIFYING VALUES AND VISION: WHERE IS NURSING GOING AND WHY?

In the first three chapters, we covered many aspects of the nursing crises and discussed other influences on care. Our overriding purpose is to excite nurses toward empowered change to help set directions for care. In order to be a part of change, nurses must find their voices as individuals and then work to articulate a collectively powerful voice of care.

The goal of care is straightforward: to create optimal health across the life span while providing comfort and dignity for everyone we serve. Ensuring democratic access to those services across socioeconomic, ethnic, racial, and cultural margins and global boundaries is also part of the goal. This is why nursing does what it does. However, we have not reached that goal; thus, we are in "crisis." We must attend to the SR principles and make a forthright appraisal of where nursing is going and why. Chapters 1–3 took a historical look at where nursing has been and where it is currently, and why. The purpose of nursing is constant, but where is nursing headed in this new century?

It is all about care. A new century is a perfect time to reassert the core of nursing. You know those New Year's resolutions that we make somewhere around December 31? It feels good to think about the possibilities and to realize that we have "another chance." Well, instead of a singular new year, we have a new century to think about. The road map to care already exists; there are just more destinations, and there is more urgency to the work that we must do. As Robert Frost (1874–1963) wrote, "The woods are lovely, dark and deep, but I have promises to keep, and miles to go before I sleep" (*Stopping by Woods on a Snowy Evening*). Nursing too has promises to keep, many obstacles, and a long journey before we will fully actualize our purpose of care.

In previous chapters, we have offered many directions in nursing based on the many drivers of care—everything from reimbursement models to new diseases. We asked you to identify your values for nursing, for care. Take out those responses because you will need them to answer the questions and to follow the eight steps (if you haven't yet had a chance to write your values for nursing, don't worry; now is a perfect opportunity). Now let's design some questions and employ the eight steps of the SR process to begin developing a clear vision for nursing.

Table 7-4 is an example of the SR steps using a care objective from our vision (develop nurses' actualization of their highest vision of care to bring peace and possibility to the world's children), but please conduct this exercise using your objectives for care. You may want better employee retention, improved client satisfaction, fewer nosocomial infections, or no medication errors, or you may want to halt the AIDS epidemic in Sub-Saharan Africa. Please answer these questions using your objectives/goals for care.

Once the steps have been identified, it is typically necessary to drill down using some focused questions in order to identify more complex resource matrices (see Table 7-5). The eight steps help to bring the values and vision into sharper focus. The questions help determine if the enterprise is in alignment with the stated values and vision. Remember the values and vision that we are using for our example: *Values: empowered nursing, integrity, respect for others, cultural acceptance, peace, childhood for every child, excellence. Vision: Peace and possibility for the world's children created by nursing's actualization of its highest vision of care.* From the earlier brief example of an SR process, we can see that where nursing is and where our particular values and vision seek to go are not aligned. We have work to do!

Appendix 7 offers an example of a strategic review template created by the authors.

Table 7-4   The Eight Steps of the Strategic Review Process Using a Care Example

1. Identify the purpose of the strategic planning process; what is the objective(s) to be accomplished? *Objective: Empower nurses to find their voice to effect positive change in care.*
2. Identify SR team members. *Michele, LeAnn, and you.*
3. Identify what will be assessed. *Nurses' ability to participate in decision-making and change processes that impact care.*
4. Identify, develop, or access expertise to interpret what is discovered. *Individual team members may need to access learning materials that explain business practices, attend conferences or seminars about business practices, and/or hire a consultant to help navigate business skill needs.*
5. Interpret findings. *Through data analysis using resources such as the* Harvard Business Review, *compare what nurses currently know about business with what is identified as the basic level needed to manage the business of care.*
6. Make recommendations. *Based on the findings, focus on the strengths of, weaknesses in, opportunities of, and threats to, empowerment of nursing as a positive change agent in the business of care. Recommend classes, group activities, etc., that nurses can attend to become effective change agents.*
7. Set strategies. *Expose all nurses to the basic principles of business management.*
8. Assess strategy success. *Ultimately, nursing will be a healthy occupation that plays a strategic role in the delivery of care that impacts all of the profession, creating a worldwide change in the lives of all children. This change will be measured by the reduction in the health challenges facing children around the world. This objective is so large that we need to create smaller benchmarks to track success; an example of such a benchmark is requiring a course in business management in all BSN programs.*

Does Nursing, as a Professional Entity, Have Clear Vision?

The American Nurses Association is the self-declared leader in the establishment of nursing standards, accreditation, and certification: "ANCC is the world's largest and most prestigious nurse credentialing organization, a subsidiary of the American Nurses Association" (ANCC, 2008a). The ANA has created a vision for the ideal qualities of a hospital to which nurses will be attracted: The Magnet Recognition Program. The ANCC has also created the Pathway to Excellence Program. The program is committed to nurses—to what nurses identify as important to their practice—and values nurses' contributions in the workplace. This designation confirms to the public that nurses working in a Pathway to Excellence organization know that their efforts are supported.

Table 7-5   Example of Questions That Identify Resource Issues

1. Is this a problem-based plan (such as a quality improvement initiative), or is this plan intended to redesign structures, process, and/or governance? *Redesign of structure, processes, and governance; a complex multilevel change.*
2. What is/are the product(s) that we seek to improve? *Care.*
3. Is there financial viability? *A strengthened and healthier nursing workforce benefits all.*
4. What are the responsibilities and decision-making of involved persons and programs? *Commitment to learning, self-improvement, and expanded worldviews; decision-making will be based on principle-centered personal leadership; discipline and dedication to learning will be cardinal.*
5. What are the strategic team members' rights, responsibilities, and roles? *The ANA's Bill of Rights for Registered Nurses (ANA, 2008).*
6. How will performance be measured? *Nurse retention rates, nurse satisfaction surveys, client outcomes, expressed empowerment, and peace and possibility created through care for the world's children.*
7. Are structures aligned with purpose? *No.*
8. Are processes aligned with purpose? *No.*
9. How is communication managed within the enterprise and externally? *Fifteen million nurses are represented by an average of 4% nurse administrators, or just 2 nurse leaders/managers for every 75 nurses (Health Resources and Service Administration [HRSA], 2004). With these poor ratios, communication is not effective.*
10. What are corporate- and discipline-specific cultural considerations? *The culture of nursing has several universal characteristics: codependence, compassion, empathy, tendency to be involved with service, desire to contribute positively, enabling, victimization mentality, scarcity thinking, generosity, critical thinking, lifelong learning, tendency toward martyrdom, high stress levels related to ineffective coping, inadequate support systems and unrealistic professional expectations, multitasking, tolerance, acceptance, "eating their young," professional disconnection across and between levels of nursing and across unique nursing disciplines, female majority in the workforce (only 5.4% male; HRSA, 2004), aging (average age in 2004 was 46.8 [HRSA, 2004]), dedication, advocacy, selfless behavior, smoking habits (12% of registered nurses smoke [Schmidt, 2000]), unhealthy lifestyle choices (54% are overweight or obese [Miller et al., 2008]), and professionally admiration and respect from the public.*
11. Empirical data are "easy" to analyze; how will affective and subjective information be evaluated? *Surveys, questionnaires, interviews, and anecdotal reports.*
12. Who needs to be included (individuals, departments, consultants, management, etc.)? *Nurses at every level and across every unique discipline of care.*

(Continued)

Table 7-5   Example of Questions That Identify Resource Issues *(Continued)*

13. What are nursing's strengths? *15 million strong, care-centered, intelligent, well-educated, service-oriented, tolerant, culturally diverse members with strong work ethics focused on universality of care.*
14. What are nursing's weaknesses? *Multiple levels, poor interlevel relationships/communication, insufficient leadership, healthcare financing models that do not favor nursing, historical gender roles, multiple drivers, global issues and pressures, and poor health.*
15. What are nursing's threats? *Financial challenges in health care, population pressures, poverty, diseases/resistance, global warming and environmental ills, market competition, more attractive careers with fewer stressors and better wages and opportunities, and an aging nursing workforce.*
16. What are nursing's opportunities? *Positive empowered change, potential for growth, and nurses' actualization of their highest vision of care.*

The award "invites other nurses to join their colleagues in this desirable and nurturing environment" (ANCC, 2008b). This designation stretches beyond hospital walls and may include any setting where nurses work. These are two of the clearest visions set before nursing, but they do not fundamentally change nursing and nurses; they seek to change where nurses work.

The National League for Nursing's (NLN's) Board of Governors wrote in its 2005 position statement, *Transforming Nursing Education*, that "new models of nursing education must emerge . . . The primary drivers of transformation in nursing education are societal need . . . demand . . . [and] accountability," and "we are on the cusp of significant change in nursing education" (NLN, 2005). Although this vision is clearly directing nurse educators to "change," there is not a clear end point. What will nurse education in 2020 look like? Could you describe a 2020 school of nursing to someone who knows nothing about health care or healthcare education based on the NLN's vision?

Other visions of nursing revolve around the launching of technology in a multitude of directions. Again, this does not speak to nursing specifically; it speaks to tools of the trade. We will continue to evolve using tools. Isn't that what people have done since the dawn of man? Although it plays a role, technology does not define nursing or nurses.

The International Council of Nurses (ICN) described its vision for nursing through a mission statement:

Our mission is to lead our societies toward better health. Working together within ICN, we harness the knowledge and enthusiasm of the entire nursing profession to promote healthy lifestyles, healthy workplaces, and healthy communities. We foster the health of our societies as well as individuals by supporting strategies of sustainable development that mitigate poverty, pollution, and other underlying causes of illness. (ICN, 2008)

The ICN (2008) defined a vision statement as "a compelling image of the preferred future that sets out a group's or organization's highest aspirations in clear, powerful, confident language." This picture is a little clearer, but do you see your distinct role in this vision?

The Brigham and Women's Hospital (a teaching affiliate of Harvard Medical School) vision for nursing is stated in three tenets: excellent care to patients and families, the very best staff, and the safest environments (Brigham and Women's Hospital, 2008). This vision is not about nurses; it is about how nurses work and what the nursing setting looks like.

In 2000, the 189 member countries of the World Health Organization (WHO) adopted the Millennium Declaration. From this declaration, a "roadmap" (strategies) was created with goals intended to be reached by 2015. Table 7-6 outlines these strategies: the eight Millennium Development Goals. This is a vision that nursing can and must participate in; however, a vision for the role of nurses is not described.

At the time of this writing, public health nurses across the country are participating in the Public Health Accreditation Board's (PHAB) vetting process of the proposed 31 standards and 109 measures for local public health and 31 standards and 116 measures for state public health accreditation. Standard 5.2 B, *Engage in State or Local Health Department Strategic Planning*, includes four measures specifically targeted to strategic planning (SP) competence. PHAB is an outgrowth of the need to respond to the IOM's *The Future of the Public's*

Table 7-6   The World Health Organization's Eight Millennium Development Goals

1. Eradicate extreme poverty and hunger
2. Achieve universal primary education
3. Promote gender equality and empower women
4. Reduce child mortality
5. Improve maternal health
6. Combat HIV/AIDS, malaria, and other diseases
7. Ensure environmental sustainability
8. Develop a global partnership for development

Source: WHO, 2008.

Health, published in 2003. The response to the chasms in public health identified in their report led to the need for an accreditation process for public health. It is timely that one standard and four measures set the bar for the need to know and participate in SP!

Here is an organization that may not have hit your radar: the Space Nursing Society (SNS). "The Space Nursing Society is an international space advocacy organization devoted to space nursing and the contribution to space exploration by Registered Nurses" (SNS, 2008). There is actually a diagnostic code for injuries sustained from a spacecraft: ICD-9 code E 845. With space as the "final frontier," imagine the values and visions for nursing that can revolve around care in and of the universe (they definitely need a strategic plan)!

There are many other examples of visions for nursing; healthcare futurists abound. Visions are not futurist "Jetsons" rocketing toward a science fiction-type destiny. The NLN (2005) says it well: "We are on the cusp of significant change." However, we, as a profession, have yet to clearly communicate a clarifying and unifying vision based on articulated values that can be understood, adopted, and embraced by all nurses. Care is our product, why we do what we do. How do we direct that care for today and tomorrow? What will the picture of nursing look like in 1 year? In 5, 10, 20, and 100 years?

In their article "10 Rules for Strategic Innovators," Govindarajan and Trimble (2005) give us five sound reasons to create innovative visions for nursing, for care (Table 7-7). We can add one more to that list: heal and strengthen nursing. "Customers everywhere are empowered, and their needs are changing rapidly as they live longer in the developed world and live better in the developing world. Such changes affect . . . services" (Govindarajan & Trimble, 2005). Is nursing ready for this change?

"Where there is no vision, the people perish."
—Proverbs 29:18

Table 7-7   Five Visions for Nursing

1. Drive growth
2. Create jobs
3. Build wealth
4. Give employees [nurses] new purpose
5. Revitalize organizations

Source: Govindarajan & Trimble, 2005.

ELEMENT 3—MISSION, GOALS, AND STRATEGIC OBJECTIVES: BRINGING THOSE VALUES AND VISIONS TO LIFE

In the preceding section, we discovered several visions that sit before us. Some are external, some aspire to be wellsprings within nursing, and some are facility specific (Magnet Status) or even cross international (or universal) borders. As we journey into the heart of developing missions, goals, and objectives, we will continue to use the example of our vision of peace and possibility for the world's children, but please take the time to use an example that holds meaning for you. Like most processes, you learn better from your own experiences.

Bringing values and vision to life requires implementation strategies— methods or steps that will take us from Point A (where we are) to Point B (where we want to be). The mission is broken down into manageable objectives and goals that are further dissected into individual strategies (activities). If we try to eat the whole elephant by attempting to create peace and possibility for the world's children without an implementation plan, we will not succeed. An example closer to home would be to try to throw yourself into remodeling your kitchen without any construction experience. Chances are, you would have a pretty big mess and may even abandon the project.

Let's bring values and vision to life. Figure 7-3 is an example of the process in a flow chart.

Figure 7-3   The process flow.

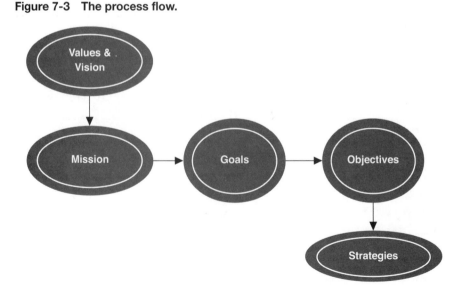

Deciding on the best implementation strategies flows from the SR; the kitchen remodel would involve learning carpentry skills, researching city codes, and acquiring the necessary equipment and learning how to operate it safely, etc. For our example, the vision is "peace and possibility," and the *mission* is to empower nurses to actualize their highest vision of care. The mission statement is the broad declaration of nursing's primary purpose for existence.

Whereas many industries have shifted their mission statement in order to survive and compete in changing economies, nursing's mission has endured across eras, generations, borders, and cultures. For example, the mission of the auto industry in the 1900s was volume production (also known as Fordism). The goal, through the use of unskilled laborers assembling inter-changeable parts, was to produce standardized goods as quickly as possible. Sound familiar? Today, divergence and environmental responsibility dominate the mission statements of most automobile manufacturers. Nursing's mission has been, is, and always will be the summative equivalent of theories, defini-tions, and concepts of a singular purpose: care.

Being clear about the "why we are here" launches the process of determin-ing the objectives and goals that we want to achieve. The mission is care; therefore, goals seek to establish benchmarks to achieve care. A popular acronym for defining goals is SMART: specific, measurable, achievable, rele-vant, and time based. Susan Heathfield (2008), a human resources specialist, suggests that SMART goals for this new millennium also include such words as *stretching, synergistic, systematic,* and *significant; meaningful, memorable,* and *motivating; action plans, accountability,* and *acumen; realistic, resonat-ing, results oriented, rewarding,* and *responsible;* and *tangible, timely,* and *thoughtful.*

Here is a timeless example, from Lewis Carroll's *Alice's Adventures in Wonderland,* of why we need goals.

"Cheshire Puss . . . would you tell me, please, which way I ought to go from here?" "That depends a good deal on where you want to get to," said the cat. "I don't much care where," said Alice. "Then it doesn't matter which way you go," said the cat. "So long as I get somewhere," Alice added as an explanation. "Oh, you're sure to do that . . . if you only walk long enough," said the cat.

Every goal should be directly linked to a core value, lest you wonder off "somewhere" with Alice. Hyrum Smith (of Franklin-Covey) developed a model for goal-setting called the "Franklin success triangle," or the "Franklin productivity pyramid" (Franklin, 1989). See Figure 7-4.

Here are some examples of goals that we have set to accomplish our vision, which is based on our values:

- Author a series of texts on strategies that empower nurses
- Develop a Web business that supports and empowers nurses (please visit http://nursesfornursesinternational.com)
- Get 200,000 nurses to read our books
- Get 500,000 nurses to join Nurses for Nurses International
- Get 500,000 nurses to work together to effect positive change in nursing to eliminate the "crisis" label.

Next, create a timeline for your goals. See Figure 7-5 for an example of our timeline.

These goals meet the SMART criteria and relate directly to our values. Also notice that some of the goals can be accomplished in a short time, whereas some require long-range planning. In addition, our goals are hierarchical. We

---

Figure 7-4   Success triangle.

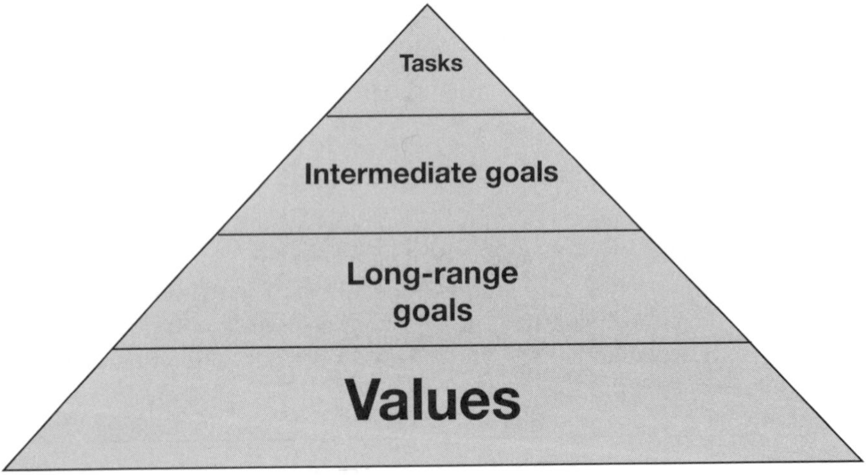

Source: Smith, 1991.

Figure 7-5   **Example of a goal timeline.**

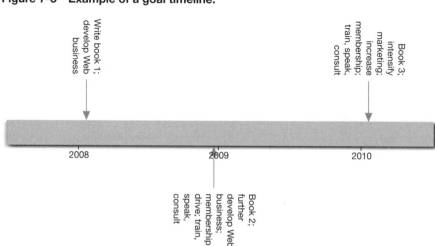

need to complete one before we can move on to the next. Please take a moment to draft the goals for your personal or professional vision that you have been considering as you wind your way through this text. Remember to make them SMART, and be sure that they flow from your values. Three to five goals usually creates plenty of work.

Goal 1: _____

Goal 2: _____

Goal 3: _____

Goal 4: _____

Goal 5: _____

Once clearly defined goals are established, objectives are set. The objectives are the "how-to" components of the goals. Recall that these objectives are not ordinary objectives; these are strategic objectives. An example of an ordinary objective for a goal of publishing a nursing textbook might be to study the publishing business in general. That may take us on a winding path to our goal

Table 7-8   Examples of Strategic Objectives

- Understand the nursing publishing industry; target the top 10 publishing houses.
- Compare and contrast available nursing texts that are related to business.
- Understand book proposal processes for various publishing houses.

of publishing a nursing text. However, a strategic objective would be to study the publishing houses that produce nursing texts. Table 7-8 lists some examples of objectives related to our goals.

These are strategic objectives for our purposes. A strategic objective is a hallmark, target, or mini-success in the larger picture of the mission and its goals. Strategic objectives are cardinal activities that help us to achieve goals. Imagine our wanting to be successful authors without knowing anything about the publishing industry.

The next step is to ask ourselves, "How do we accomplish the strategic objectives?" The methods (strategies) flow from the objectives. Project strategies can be very straightforward or very complex adventures. Change processes that involve a paradigm shift that requires a new way of thinking and problem-solving typically require more attention to multiple details. See Table 7-9 for examples of strategies we created in order to compare and contrast nursing texts related to business.

If you are an author, you may have some other strategies that have facilitated your publishing success. As you can see, these strategies are specific action steps that led to the accomplishment of our goal.

Table 7-9   Strategy Examples for Comparing Nursing Business Texts

- Visit 10 university bookstores to review texts.
- Conduct an online search of nursing texts related to business.
- Conduct a search of texts promoted by national and international nursing organizations.
- Visit public bookstores in at least three states to determine how book reps stock shelves.
- Read at least 10 current books on nursing business and/or business.

> *"The tragedy in life doesn't lie in not reaching your goal.*
> *The tragedy lies in having no goal to reach."*
> —Dr. Benjamin E. Mays, 1895–1984

Think of the mission as the big picture, the goals as sections of the big picture, the objectives as portions of those sections, and the strategies as the individual pieces that complete the picture. Strategies are the operational definitions of how the work will be accomplished.

The Architect, Change Agent, and Communicator: Three Crucial Roles in Strategic Planning

We are borrowing the team concepts created by Robert S. Kaplan and David P. Norton for the Balanced Scorecard. Kaplan and Norton (1996) identified three crucial roles in the strategic planning process: architect, change agent, and communicator.

In a general strategic plan, the architect is responsible for designing the plan based on the findings of the strategic review. The architect may be one person or a group, depending on the scope of the project. Architects create the "blueprint" that leads the process. A blueprint shows the rooms but does not furnish and decorate; that is the job of the change agents. Change agents are the "builders" of the plan. They are the motivators who implement the new strategies. The "communicator" keeps all the dots connected. This is the "strategic engineer," or liaison, who keeps the project front and center. The communicator is a master at team processes, synergy, and collaboration. The communicator has another tough job: achieving buy-in and support from all stakeholders. See Table 7-10 for the job descriptions of a strategic planning team.

This chapter took the previously discussed challenges facing nursing and applied key elements of strategic planning processes to them. The SR can be

Remember—No nurse left behind. It takes a village to achieve strategic alignment from top to bottom. All nurses, across the many levels and borders of nursing, are vital to the profession of care.

Table 7-10   Roles and Responsibilities of a Strategic Planning Team

Team Member/Role	Responsibilities and Characteristics
Strategic Review Committee Nursing Leadership & Management	Set direction based on best practices and the strategic review; articulate clear values and vision; effectively utilize resources; build capacity; allocate and manage resources responsibly; align process with standards, guidelines, and ethics; empower professional growth of all; set the climate and culture for change.
Strategic Planning Task Force(s) Architect(s)	Display planning competence; consult with stakeholders; establish goals, objectives, strategies, and evaluation criteria; employ a clear understanding of quality improvement processes.
Strategic Planning Team Change Agents	Master change processes and theory; show an understanding of human behaviors and the strategic planning process; motivate others; involve all stakeholders; perform competent conflict resolution; use effective communication—written and verbal.
Strategic Engineer/ Liaison Communicator	Practice skilled communication; display an expert understanding of change processes and theories and of strategic planning; possess values and vision aligned with the enterprise; show commitment to total quality improvement methods and strategies.

painful or rejuvenating, but it should always be respectful of people. Values should be at the heart of all that you do personally and professionally. The vision of what you want in your professional or personal life is solidly founded in your values. What you do—your mission—flows from that vision. Three key roles in a strategic planning process are architects, change agents, and communicators. Building a team facilitates success.

In Section 1, we covered the need for the tenets of business and strategic planning in nursing. In Section 2, we discussed the principles and foundations of strategic planning. In Section 3, we will dig deeper to understand the theories and rationale behind this business construct. Before we move on, we have included some examples of how nurse leaders have employed the axioms of strategic planning to improve care in a world of nursing that is bombarded by a multitude of drivers and influences.

THREE CASE STUDIES DEMONSTRATING HOW SP IS APPLIED BY PRACTICING NURSES TO SOLVE PROBLEMS IN THEIR SPECIALTY AREAS IN NURSING

CASE STUDY #1:

Where Are We? Where Do We Want to Be? How Do We Get There?

Julie A. Serstad, MSN, RN

The challenges of a new position are almost always exciting if you view the glass half full, as I do. I usually sit back for a while, maybe 3–6 months, to listen and learn about the agency, structure, employees, informal communication, etc.

My arrival at my most recent position as the director of Health Services for a large local health department was no different. It's what we all do when we meet a new client, go to a new neighborhood, and perform an assessment. The nursing process becomes a part of all that we do.

One of my first observations was that there was no specific strategic plan in place. I felt that the staff had a strong commitment to the work being done, but no direction or vision. I approached my supervisor with a plan and a request for an outside facilitator to conduct a formal strategic planning workshop for us. I also requested funding to hold the session at an off-site facility. I was given the go-ahead.

It is so vital to have the support and encouragement of management for a strategic plan to be successful. This includes upper and middle management. Many of the direct line staff were very skeptical and hesitant about participating, so meeting with supervisors before informing the staff was very important. I shared information on the value of strategic planning with the supervisors. This was to be the first "all staff" strategic planning meeting that most of the staff had ever experienced. I also required all staff to attend.

Our session objectives included:

1. Review of Health Services progress and achievements in the last 12 months.
2. Explore and discuss important factors in the external and internal operating environment to establish a realistic context for discussion and planning.
3. Describe and commit to a proactive and realistic future scenario for departments within Health Services and establish a 3-year strategic framework to support that vision.

The first two objectives are basically an assessment of the organization. We identified a framework, based on a scale from 1 to 10 (10 being the most positive), and listed the characteristics of a program at the 1–3 level, 4–6 level, 7–8 level, and 9–10 level. Then we explored our current operating environment. Participants identified the trends, issues, and influences as pertinent factors in our current environment.

We identified a strategic framework by developing our mission statement, our vision statement, and then strategic goals for the organization as a whole. We realized the importance of recognizing each division's individual strategies and so separated into those divisions and listed services and success indicators.

We came to consensus on our overall strategic goals, and the three separate areas did the same for their individual strategic goals for the next 12–36 months. We made a commitment to revisit the organizational goals and strategies at least yearly, and the individual area goals on a quarterly basis.

The involvement and participation of the entire team is critical to buy-in and to the success of a strategic plan. This highlights the importance of choosing your facilitator very carefully. The plan is not a static process, but rather a living, viable series of actions that will be revised and have new solutions over time. The value of embracing a comprehensive plan cannot be overemphasized because it truly sets the stage for excellence in practice and assurance of protection and sustainability of the public's health.

CASE STUDY #2:

Why Strategic Planning: Meeting Challenges in Frontier Health Care

Peggy Stevens, BSN, RN

Public health nursing in a frontier community poses many challenges. The community itself provides challenges, with isolation, lack of services, and a depressed economy. Limited financial, facility, and equipment resources are challenging enough, but added to these dilemmas and barriers to care is the shortage in the public health nurse (PHN) workforce; not only is staffing a problem, but funding programs and having competitive salaries is a tremendous problem as well.

Creating a clear set of strategies based on thoughtful planning is the only way to figure out how to provide care in resource-challenged settings. So, one has to be creative. First, I think that one has to determine the community's needs—what services are most needed—and align those needs with available funding sources.

Finding funding sources to help offset costs is where strategic planning is a really helpful tool. Frontier communities have very few financial resources. Small counties must depend on outside funding sources just to pay basic wages and provide basic services (like immunizations, Women Infant and Children [WIC], and epidemiology). Clear implementation strategies are necessary lest grants drive care.

Developing budgets, finding funding sources, managing a workforce, being a "jack-of-all-trades," and implementing quality measures is a tough job when one or two people—part time—have to make everything work. Strategic planning helps us to keep on track and make the best use of funding, programs, and people while trying to meet the many healthcare needs of our community.

CASE STUDY #3:

Strategic Planning in Acute Care Settings

Carrie Stensrud, BSN, RN, CCRN-CSC

The Bitterroot Chapter is a small, local affiliation of the American Association of Critical Care Nurses. Despite the fact that we are the only connection to our national organization in our region, we failed to have active participation from the critical care nurses in our immediate and surrounding areas. Subsequently, we were challenged by a lack of direction and purpose. We struggled with recruiting and maintaining active chapter members. In order to address these issues, we voted to hire a professional consultant to streamline our efforts, revive the floundering chapter, and develop a strategic plan.

The chapter reviewed strategic plans of similar organizations on a national and regional level. We reviewed the mission, vision, and values of our national organization and brainstormed how we wanted our chapter to look in the future. We met with our consultant, and board members were given the task of identifying the reasons for planning and designing a process to meet the needs of the chapter. We assessed and evaluated our chapter by reviewing our history and prior accomplishments, articulating our previous and current strategies, identifying our internal and external stakeholders, and reviewing the effectiveness of our current programs. After summarizing the information collected, it was time to make sense of the data and agree upon our priorities.

Our strategic plan is heavily weighted on recruitment and retention, but also includes plans to increase the vendor support at our annual Critical Care Symposium, launch a significant community service project, and establish a scholarship fund. Our plan is meant to be a work in progress, a reference document that clearly states our goals but can also be amended by the needs of our chapter. We focused on making our goals attainable in a 3–5 year timeline and did not try to exceed realistic expectations. By having our goals so specific and reasonable, we are set up for success and find ourselves already celebrating those successes.

We now have mission and vision statements to guide our work. We have clearly defined short- and long-term goals regarding recruitment and retention, growth strategies, future programs, and benefits to our members. Our strategic planning process has given us a sense of direction and a renewed energy for providing leadership and educational opportunities to our colleagues and a level of excellence in critical care to our patients and their families.

REVIEW QUESTIONS

1. A strategic review also may be referred to as what?
2. What are the three main components of a SR?
3. SR is comparative to what part of the nursing process?
4. How do values and vision impact SR?
5. In Susan Heathfield's version, what does the acronym SMART stand for?
6. List the three crucial roles in the SR process.

REFERENCES

Altman, L. (2000, March 24). Study links bacteria, long nails and baby deaths. *The New York Times*. Retrieved April 29, 2009, from http://www.nytimes.com/2000/03/24/us/study-links-bacteria-long-nails-and-baby-deaths.html

American Nurses Association (ANA). (2008). *The ANA's bill of rights for registered nurses*. Silver Spring, MD: Author.

American Nurses Credentialing Center (ANCC). (2008a). *Accreditation of continuing nursing education providers*. Retrieved December 1, 2008, from http://www.nursing credentialing.org/ContinuingEducation/Accreditation.aspx

American Nurses Credentialing Center (ANCC). (2008b). *Program overview announcing the Pathway to Excellence™ Program.* Retrieved December 1, 2008, from http://www.nursingcredentialing.org/Pathway/ProgramOverview.aspx

Brigham and Women's Hospital. (2008). *Vision for Nursing at BWH.* Retrieved December 1, 2008, from http://www.brighamandwomens.org/nursing/BWHNursingVision.aspx

Govindarajan, V., & Trimble, C. (2005). *10 rules for strategic innovators.* Boston: Harvard Business School Press.

Health Resources and Services Administration (HRSA). (2008). *The registered nurse population: Findings from the National Sample Survey of Registered Nurses.* Retrieved December 1, 2008, from http://bhpr.hrsa.gov/healthworkforce/reports/nursing/samplesurvey00/default.htm

Heathfield, S. (2008). *Beyond traditional SMART goals.* Retrieved December 3, 2008, from http://www.humanresources.about.com/cs/performancemanage/a/goalsetting.htm

International Council of Nursing (ICN). (2008). *ICN's vision for the future of nursing.* Retrieved December 1, 2008, from http://www.icn.ch/visionstatement.htm

Kaplan, R. S., & Norton, D. P. (1996). *The Balanced Scorecard: Translating strategy into action.* Boston: Harvard Business School Press.

Miller, S. K., Alpert, P. T., & Cross, C. L. (2008). Overweight and obesity in nurses, advanced practice nurses, and nurse educators. *Journal of the American Academy of Nurse Practitioners, 20*(5), 259–265.

Moolenaar, R. L., Crutcher, J. M., San Joaquin, V. H., Sewell, L. V., Hutwagner, L. C., Carson, L. A., et al. (2000). A prolonged outbreak of *Pseudomonas aeruginosa* in a neonatal intensive care unit: Did staff fingernails play a role in disease transmission? *Infection Control and Hospital Epidemiology, 21*(2), 80–85.

Mosby's dictionary of medicine, nursing and health professions (7th ed.). (2005). St. Louis, MO: Mosby Elsevier.

National League for Nursing (NLN). (2004). *Mission and goals.* Retrieved November 28, 2008, from http://www.nln.org/aboutnln/ourmission.htm

National League for Nursing (NLN). (2005). *Position statement: Transforming nursing education.* Retrieved November 28, 2008, from http://www.nln.org

Schmidt, E. (2008, November 12). UCLA study reveals smoking's effects on nurses' health, death rates. *UCLANews.* Retrieved December 1, 2008, http://www.newsroom.ucla.edu/portal/ucla/PRN-new-ucla-study-reveals-smoking-71590.aspx

Smith, H. (1989). *Franklin Day Planner System.* Salt Lake City, UT: Franklin International Insti-tute, Inc.

Space Nursing Society. (2008). *About Space Nursing.* Retrieved April 29, 2009, from http://www.spacenursingsociety.net

World Health Organization (WHO). (2000). *Health and Millennium Development Goals.* Retrieved December 1, 2008, from http://www.who.int/mdg

Sample Template of the Strategic Planning Process

Nursing's Strategic Planning Worksheet:

Rate the following resources from 1 to 5: 1= *not essential*; 2 = *nice to have*; 3 = *somewhat essential*; 4 = *beneficial/mostly essential*; 5 = *essential*

a. People _____

b. Money _____

c. Knowledge/expertise _____

d. Relationships/team _____

e. Partnerships _____

f. Learning opportunities/schools _____

g. Technology _____

h. Equipment _____

i. Time _____

j. Other _____

Now rate each of the above by (*your*) priority (1–5):

a. People _____

b. Money _____

c. Knowledge/expertise _____

d. Relationships/team _____

e. Partnerships _____

f. Learning opportunities/schools _____

g. Technology _____

h. Equipment _____

i. Time _____

j. Other _____

Ask the following questions:

   a. What is the purpose of the strategic planning process? What is/are the objective(s) to be accomplished?

   b. Who will the strategic review team members be?

   c. What will be assessed?

   d. How will we identify, develop, or access expertise to interpret what is discovered?

   e. How will we interpret findings?

   f. Based on the findings, who will be responsible for making recommendations (with a focus on the strengths, weaknesses, opportunities, and threats to nursing empowerment)?

   g. Which strategies will be used and how?

   h. How will the strategies be prioritized?

   i. How will we assess strategy success (evaluation)?

PART 3

Architects, Change Agents, and Communicators: Digging a Little Deeper

CHAPTER 8

Overview of Strategic Planning Theories: Strategic Planning Architecture

─────── **OBJECTIVES** ───────

1. Identify three business theories.
2. Identify similarities between nursing theory and business theory.
3. Describe how SP architects are like a GPS locator.
4. Summarize business theorists and how their ideas can be applied by nursing.
5. Identify the tasks of the SP architect.
6. Describe how scalability applies to the SP process.
7. Evaluate visions for nursing from a variety of professional organizations.
8. Identify tools for obtainable goals that relate to the desired vision and values.
9. Distinguish the roles needed to create and implement a strategic plan.

Many leaders (and ideas) in businesses have paved the path of knowledge for the enterprise functions of business. Leaders such as Porter, Kaplan, Norton, and Drucker and ideas like SWOT, risk identification, and project management give us the necessary tools to understand the theory behind strategic planning. There are many models and theories in both nursing and in business, which can leave any reader reeling from cognitive overload. At a glance, these models and theories may seem diametrically opposed, creating an "us" and a "them." environment. This chapter offers the reader a view to understand the theory behind the principles of strategic planning and demonstrates the universal compatibility of two seemingly diametric paradigms. Although necessary, theory can be tedious. To combat this arduous material, the chapter concludes with some fun. Readers will have the opportunity to "imagineer" care through preliminary synthesis of models and theories from business and nursing.

STRATEGIC PLANNING ARCHITECTS

How do we create new and contemporary (architectural) designs of care? Let's say that it is your job to design a green (environmentally responsive) hospital. Where would you begin, what would you need to know, and, as the architect, what tasks would you need to complete? Before starting the project, you would need to be expert in environmental engineering, resource capabilities, construction, and materials. From there, you would design a blueprint for construction that gives instructions to the builders and describes the quality and types of materials, building codes, and specifications.

Architects of strategic planning decide where to begin. They define the needs and tasks necessary to build a sustainable plan. Kaplan and Norton (*The Balanced Scorecard*) portrayed a change management team that has three key roles: architect, change agent, and communicator (Kaplan & Norton, 1996). Architects have a thorough understanding of the values, vision, and mission. Strategic architects understand the new focus of the strategic planning (SP), but most important, they understand the theories that drive the need for an SP process. The role of an architect in the SP process is to give instructions (a blueprint with clear objectives) that will guide the personnel and facilitate appropriate implementation based on the type of setting. For example, a long-term care facility will have unique personnel needs (the average nurse-to-client ratio is 1:40) that the blueprint must consider. The long-term care setting is based on labor-intensive practices, such as dependent human movement and care, that are designed for physical functioning of residents and not for optimal nursing care efficiency. Compare this to an ICU, where every amenity is efficiently close to the patient and readily accessible to the nurse—two very different blueprints for nursing care.

The architect has a vital understanding of the profession. A profession is founded on theories that guide the conventions of the vocation. Every discipline has guiding operational theories that direct its practice. Professional nursing originates in theory. Nursing theory is the body of knowledge that supports and directs professional nursing practice. Theory knowledge is a main element of the SP architect's toolkit.

THEORIES: GPS LOCATORS NAVIGATING THE WINDING PATHS OF CHANGE

How have you reacted to nursing theories in your previous studies? Do you have a favorite theorist? Or do you shy away from or avoid theories? Nursing does not corner the market on theory. Many professions and vocations are, like nursing, theory laden. The nursing process did not originate from nursing;

it actually comes from the social sciences. Likewise, theories have been adapted from other disciplines and used as tools to "professionalize" the profession. For example, Madeline Leininger's *Transcultural Nursing Theory* is based on the study of anthropology. That which cannot be explained and justified cannot be reimbursed or advanced. Theories are the architectural design that gives form to professions, thus the blueprints.

Theories can seem confusing and cumbersome unless their process is understood. They are simply well-considered, substantiated, and organized systems of current knowledge that offer meaning. There are three levels to this system: theories, models, and frameworks. Theories are more detailed than models, and models in turn are more detailed than frameworks. The overarching purpose of all three is to define and explain observable occurrences such as care. They also strive to interpret occurrences in terms that are professionally relevant, explaining them so that everyone in the profession understands.

For example, care occurs in every culture and country, so it is a universal phenomenon. Can you define, describe, and then interpret care, including the multitude of traditions, beliefs, behaviors, and practices that encapsulate it? We are surrounded by human caring—quality, spiritual, physical, intensive, empathetic, environmental, long-term, and emergent care (just to name a few types). There are also all the forms of care as an affective characteristic, such as nurturing, protective, and cultural demonstrations of care. So, can you offer a clear summary of everything there is to know about care? Probably not, and that is OK; that's why there are theorists. The researchers dig deeper to offer a clear understanding of why things are the way they are. Theorists take a question several steps further. They hold these suppositions up to the light and ask who, what, where, when, why, and how.

Recall the theory that bloodletting was a good treatment. George Washington was a believer. Suffering from hoarseness and a sore throat, he directed the gentleman who oversaw his estate to conduct venesection (one technique of bloodletting). Three physicians attended to President Washington in the last days of his life and took turns bloodletting—not to mention administering an assortment of vinegar, molasses, poultices, and balms, and soaking his feet in hot water—as a means to cure him of his cold (he had been healthy prior to catching the cold). President Washington "was a strong believer in bloodletting, having used it successfully to cure various maladies affecting his Negro slaves" (Vadakan, 2002). Bloodletting of 20–40 ounces (the equivalent to approximately four units of blood) was performed on President Washington at least 5 times in fewer than 2 days. Interestingly enough, the original First Lady, Martha Washington, did not believe in bloodletting—perhaps a more scientific mind?

There were various definitions and explanations justifying why some people improved with bloodletting, but the practice was founded in "magic and religious ceremonies" (Seigworth, 2002). For more than 3000 years, for lack of a good theorist, bloodletting was a common practice.

Theorists not only define and explain, but they also justify. Imagine trying to define, explain, and justify bloodletting using current knowledge. Theories are based on evidence and principles of the scientific processes.[1] Bloodletting and other practices based on beliefs and casual observations led to a need for rigorous and substantiated research. From research flows new ways of seeing and perceiving phenomena; for example, people did not always get better from bloodletting, leading someone to ask, "Are there other variables and considerations that lead to healing?"

Theories are truth seeking. Not unlike the discovery phase (strategic review) of the strategic planning process, theories gather and analyze internal and external data to create a picture of current reality. Today, there are physicians who employ bloodletting as a treatment for chronic obstructive pulmonary disease (COPD); the rationale is that bloodletting decreases red blood cells in those individuals for whom polycythemia is a complication of the disease. Other theories (as yet unsubstantiated) that prescribe bloodletting for COPD cite a decrease in oxidative stress that reduces airway inflammation (Lagente, Planquois, Leclerc, Schmidlin, & Bertrand, 2007). Theories supporting or negating the advantages of bloodletting continue to evolve as new information is discovered.

Florence Nightingale based her definitions and explanations of nursing on observations of the effects of fresh air, light, and a clean environment (including cleaning surfaces between patient use) on the decrease in infections and improved patient recovery. Her book *Notes on Nursing: What It Is and What It Is Not*, published in 1860, interprets and summarizes what she learned to be true about care. Since Florence Nightingale, purported to be the first nurse theorist (she created a theoretical framework), theories in nursing have traversed

---

[1]The process tool that makes sense of what is observed or experienced, that establishes definitions, that makes assumptions, that forms concepts and hypotheses, and that creates theoretical models is the scientific method. Regardless of discipline, the scientific method is the standard for any credible research in today's science, social, business, or philosophical avocation. Although the scientific method is not a recipe, there are at least six elements:

1. Purpose—why are we looking at this?
2. Research—quantitative and/or qualitative
3. Hypothesis—predicting the answer based on the research
4. Experiment—confirm or disprove the hypothesis
5. Analysis—record what happened during the experiment
6. Conclusion—was the hypothesis correct?

three main focal areas: industrial worker model, biomedical or medical model, and social model.

We've discussed the former industrial role of the nurse as a physician's handmaiden. Although not a theory-driven era in nursing, nonetheless it continues to influence nursing culture and societal roles. The era lasted until the mid-1900s.

The second focus of theories that led nursing was based on the biomedical model, also referred to as the medical model, which studied people as a disease or disease set. These theories continue to have great influence on nursing practice.

Finally, the third and more contemporary theory is based on social models and focuses on the patient as a whole instead of on a disease. This holistic model considers all aspects of life: culture, religion, ethnicity, gender, age, family, community, education, and life experiences. Each era of theory contributes to nursing practice in different ways depending on the academic degree or credential and age of the nurse, the practice setting, professional experiences, and management style.

What if we now add a 21st-century theory set that empowers the profession of nursing by combining traditional nursing theory with business theory? What would that look like? We are proposing that it is time for an epoch change in nursing theory. To claim the lead in care, nursing needs theories that define nurses as autonomous change agents and leaders. The industry, medical, and holistic models speak to how nurses interact with patients, medical teams, and the environment. Nursing now needs models and theories that describe how nurses interact with each other, influence care, and become global healthcare change agents. This will be the job of the SP architects.

To expand on the new theory, model, and framework, think about a global positioning system (GPS) locator. GPS locators need three satellites to triangulate[2] a specific location on Earth. One satellite provides insufficient information; divergent views are required to set a course. GPS locators use signals from 24 to 32 different satellites to help the user navigate.

Nursing has expanded its worldview over the past decades but continues to operate from insufficient information. In the same way, nurses now need to access more satellites to more accurately guide their future. An expanded worldview will strengthen nursing as we navigate a new century of care. Nursing must learn to align business models with care models.

---

[2]A trigonometric equation that uses angles from known distances (such as satellite positions) to determine a fixed point.

HOW DO BUSINESS MODELS AND THEORIES ALIGN WITH NURSING'S MODELS AND THEORIES?

Sister Callista Roy, Margaret Newman, Patricia Benner, Martha Rogers, Madeline Leininger, Virginia Henderson, Imogene King, Dorothea Orem, and Ida Jean Orlando are some of the leading nurse theorists whose names you may recognize. From Benner's simple-to-complex view of skill acquisition to Leininger's theory defining human care within the context of culture, nursing models and theories cover a wide range of nursing characteristics. Figure 8-1a offers a basic overview of some of these theorists and their work.

But who are the business theorists? The list is considerably longer than the 20 or so nursing theorists. Business theorists have defined and explained concepts in leadership, management, time, personnel, scientific management, organizational management, operations, systems, strategy, organizational psychology, and many more tenets of business. Figure 8-1b displays the contributions from four of today's leading business theorists.

Figure 8-1a   Nursing theorists and their contributions.

Theorist	Theory or Model
Sister Callista Roy	Adaptation Model
Margaret A. Newman	Health as Expanding Consciousness
Madeline Leininger	Transcultural Nursing Model
Imogene King	General Systems Theory

Figure 8-1b   Business theorists and their contributions.

Theorist(s)	Theory or Model
Robert Kaplan and David Norton	Balanced Scorecard
Michael Porter	Five Forces
Peter Drucker	Management by Objectives; father of modern management; coined the term *knowledge worker*
Taiichi Ohno	Toyota Production System

It is not our supposition that nursing and business theories are interchangeable, but there are some fundamental principles that create the underpinnings of any theory. Let's start by taking a look at the seven basic components of theory (Table 8-1).

Our next step is to compare a business problem with a nursing problem using an affinity diagram (Table 8-2). Studying the basic affinity diagram reveals how closely aligned the purposes of (healthcare) business and nursing really are.

As we build the premise that business and nursing theories must align, let's review the two main parts of strategic planning theory: design and execution. We begin with an elemental overview, highlighting the components of strategic planning and the architect's role in creating the design (Figure 8-2).

Table 8-3 uses the affinity diagram (Table 8-2) to show the architect's integration of theory with the SP.

Table 8-1 Seven Basic Components of Theory

1. Observation is made.
2. Observation or experience is explained and defined—*Bloodletting makes people well by draining out bad blood.*
3. Assumptions are made—*Blood that is bad is best drained from the body.*
4. Supporting concepts are formed—*Evil spirits cause illness; blood is the predominant humour (medieval term for the four basic body fluids; yellow bile, black bile, and phlegm are the others); imbalance in any of the four basic body humours causes disease.*
5. Develop hypothesis—*Early medical practice was based on the notion that all health matters were related to the four basic body fluids, or humours, which must be maintained in a balance at all times. Because blood is the predominant body fluid, it was hypothesized that its removal during illness helped to restore balance and therefore health.*
6. Theoretical model describing the relationships between components that lead to the observation is developed—*The theory that bloodletting was a therapeutic tool has its origins as far back as the Ancient Egyptian times; the rigors of the current scientific method were not adapted by the scientific community until the late 19th and early 20th centuries. Had President Washington lived in the 1930s, he would not have died from exsanguination.*
7. Theory is researched until diligence has been accomplished.

Table 8-2 Affinity Diagram: Business Problem and Nursing Problem Application to "Seven Components of Theory"

Problem	Make Sense of Observed or Experienced	Observations—Experience Explained/ Defined	Assumptions Made	Concepts Formed	Hypothesis Developed	Theoretical Model Constructed	Evaluation and Further Development
Loss of revenue (business)	Expenses exceed profits	Complication post-CABG* cost $20,000 and add 6–7 hospital days**	Fewer complications = cost savings	Post-op ARDS*** most common; septicemia second most common	Improved pre-, peri-, and postoperative care will decrease complications	SWOT analysis to implement quality improvement	Outcome measured post-CABG*
Complications post-CABG* (nursing)	13.64% of CABG patients experience complications (2005)**	CABG* patients are high acuity, requiring skilled intensive caregivers and environment	High rates (13.64%) of complications are related to ratio of and skill of intensive caregivers and/ or environment	Safe staffing ratios, biomedical support, and training are necessary	Decreased nurse:patient ratios and better biomedical support will decrease complications	Nurse staffing rates and patient mortality and morbidity****	Evaluate patient outcomes post-CABG*

*CABG = Coronary Artery Bypass Graft

**Cardiac Data Solutions, 2008. http://www.examhealth.com/80/23141.html

***ARDS = Adult Respiratory Distress Syndrome

****Aiken, Clarke, Sloane, Sochalski, & Silber, 2002.

Figure 8-2 Overview of the strategic planning process.

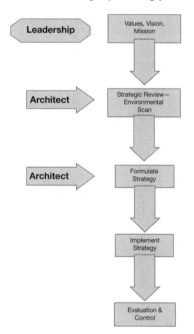

THE BASIC PRINCIPLES OF STRATEGIC PLANNING

For the purposes of this text, we have chosen to summarize Harvard Business School professor Michael Porter's "Five Forces" and "generic strategies." We are also using Kaplan and Norton's "Balanced Scorecard." Harvard professor and Palladium Group (PCI) founder Robert Kaplan and director David Norton are leaders in the development of theories of strategic planning. Porter's models and theories focus on the crafting of strategic plans, whereas those of Kaplan and Norton lean toward execution and evaluation.

Both apply theories over a period of time. This is referred to as a *business cycle*. In general, a business cycle has four stages: expansion, growth, contraction, and recession. Business cycles are dependent on business types. Individual businesses within an enterprise have unique business cycles. For example, in a busy emergency department (ED), the staff expects an increase in alcohol-related vehicular trauma on weekends and holidays and after popular local events. The influx of high-acuity patients on the weekends affects the

Table 8-3 Architect Draws from Theory to Implement the Strategic Plan

Problem	Make Sense of Observed or Experienced	Observations— Experience Explained/ Defined	Assumptions Made	Concepts Formed	Hypothesis Developed	Theoretical Model Constructed	Evaluation and Further Development
Loss of revenue (business)	Expenses exceed profits	Complication post-CABG* cost $20,000 and add 6–7 hospital days**	Fewer complications = cost savings	Post-op ARDS*** most common; septicemia second most common	Improved pre-, peri-, and postoperative care will decrease complications	SWOT analysis to implement quality improvement	Outcome measured post-CABG*
Complications post-CABG* (nursing)	13.64% of CABG patients experience complications (2005)**	CABG* patients are high acuity, requiring skilled intensive caregivers and environment	High rates (13.64%) of complications are related to ratio of and skill of intensive caregivers and/ or environment	Safe staffing ratios, biomedical support, and training are necessary	Decreased nurse:patient ratios and better biomedical support will decrease complications	Nurse staffing rates and patient mortality and morbidity****	Evaluate patient outcomes post-CABG*

Architect → Architect → Architect → Architect → Architect

*CABG = Coronary Artery Bypass Graft
**Cardiac Data Solutions, 2008. http://www.examhealth.com/80/23141.html
***ARDS = Adult Respiratory Distress Syndrome
****Aiken, Clarke, Sloane, Sochalski, & Silber, 2002.

ED business cycle. In another example, clinic nurses see an increase in business (patient visits) during influenza season. In both cases equipment and staffing needs vary with the fluctuations. Competent managers are skilled in budgeting, staffing, and equipment management in anticipation of these business cycles. Please see Table 8-4 for a detailed example of the business cycle in an ED.

The business cycle also includes normal fluctuations in an organization's economic activity. Health care's business cycles face "unique challenges and requirements . . . the healthcare industry is stressed to its limits: increasing regulations and insatiable demands for innovation, testing and risk management" (Tatum, LLC, 2008). Unstable business cycles have dominated health care since the Balanced Budget Act of 1997 (refer to Chapter 3). As nurses learn about the business of health care, it is likely that they will gain an appreciation of, and respect for, healthcare managers. Health care is one of the most complex, unpredictable, and heavily regulated business entities in existence. There is an adage in long-term care (LTC) management that they are more

Table 8-4   Example of an Emergency Department (ED) Business Cycle

Cycle	Examples
Expansion	Increase ED capacity to 40 beds—new construction; recruit 10 ED hospitalists, 20 full-time equivalent ED RNs, 5 healthcare aides, and 5 RT; acquisition of necessary supportive biomedical equipment; align with human resources and CFO
Growth	Increased ED visits over FY (fiscal year) by 28%
Contraction	Competing ED capturing 5% of ED visits; staff retention rates decreasing; loan payments versus return on investment decreasing, etc.
Recession	Demographic and sociopolitical shift in community leads to higher numbers of uninsured clientele; CMS reimbursement rates decrease with advent of "never events"; unionized staff demanding higher cost of living increase

heavily regulated than the nuclear waste industry! Regardless of whether this is true, health care is a tough business to manage. The application of business theories such as the Balanced Scorecard and the Five Forces to the challenges facing health care facilitates problem-solving and profitability. Can you identify the four stages of business cycles (expansion, growth, contraction, and recession) in your organization or practice?

The business theory of Kaplan and Norton's Balanced Scorecard theory has been rigorously tested since its publication in 1996. As a strategy tool, their management system helps organizations set strategic goals, allocate resources, set priorities for process tasks (operations), and evaluate progress and strategy effectiveness. As its title suggests, the purpose of the Balanced Scorecard is to balance all these variables. Can you imagine having clear strategic goals without the necessary support resources—for example, working on a strategy that completes a new outpatient clinic without ensuring that the door width accommodates stretchers? Or, imagine failing to track a plan's progress, only to find out that the project is completed, and no one knew when it was in the final stages. The Balanced Scorecard builds a management system that supports not only the strategies but also the necessary day-to-day operations. Figure 8-3 demonstrates the components of the Balanced Scorecard.

Now, let's apply this balanced approach to the ED example. Review Figure 8-4 for an example of necessary variables (balances) for an ED's sustainability. The point of a scorecard is to track progress in the four management process areas: financial, customer, business/operational, and learning/growth. It is a holistic view of process and change management. The Balanced Scorecard is used in a variety of organizations ranging from rural hospitals to Fortune 500 companies.[3] The transferable principles necessitate collaborative, integrated partnerships within the organization and the community. Although the doors to our units or offices close behind us as we come or go, we nurses do not work in a vacuum. Think again about Figure 8-4 and consider what parts of the cycle nursing contributes to; also consider what areas we have neglected and/or avoided, and the areas in which we have surrendered influence. Egocentrism leads any discipline into a limited worldview. The Balanced Scorecard enables all stakeholders to assess the bigger picture and support the need for metaleadership.

Michael Porter's Five Forces and generic strategies are business theories that clarify the key issues faced by a business. Recall that in the bloodletting example, what we think the problem is may or may not be accurate. The purpose of Michael Porter's Five Forces (Table 8-5) is to help discover "why things are as they are" or an in-depth strategic analysis.

---

[3]Published by *Fortune* magazine, an annual list of the top 500 U.S. companies that produce the greatest revenues.

Figure 8-3 Kaplan and Norton's Balanced Scorecard approach "balances" all fundamental variables necessary for project success.

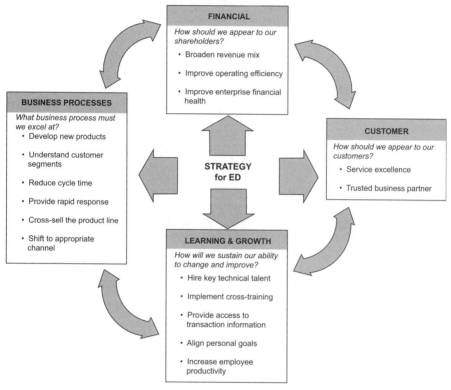

Source: Kaplan and Norton, 1996.

The Five Forces facilitate and inform the strategic review process (environmental scan, situational analysis). Because these terms do not resemble nursing theories, let's try to make sense of them. Figure 8-5 offers an example of the Five Forces applied to the ED example. These are the tools necessary for internal and external review in the strategic planning process. Rivalry is based on the competition-drives-profits economic model. Health care is a business, and all businesses seek to attain competitive advantage (customer share, high profit, recruiting and retaining the highest quality personnel, high stock performance, etc.). The other four forces determine the extent to which an enterprise (business) is able to attain the advantage.[4]

---

[4]To learn more about Michael Porter's Five Forces, visit http://porter.multimedia.hbr.org.

Figure 8-4   Balanced Scorecard template applied to an ED change.

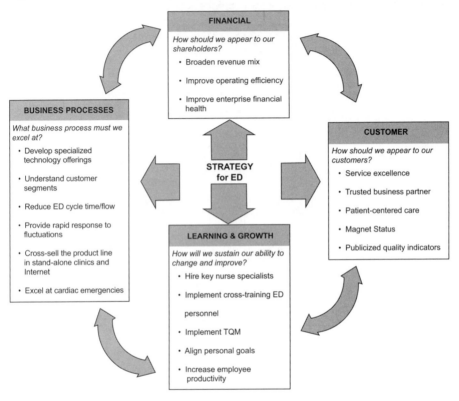

Table 8-5   Michael Porter's Five Forces

1. Supplier power
2. Barriers to entry
3. Buyer power
4. Threat of substitutes
5. Rivalry

Figure 8-5   Michael Porter's Five Forces: A basic application to analyze current internal and external factors affecting an ED.

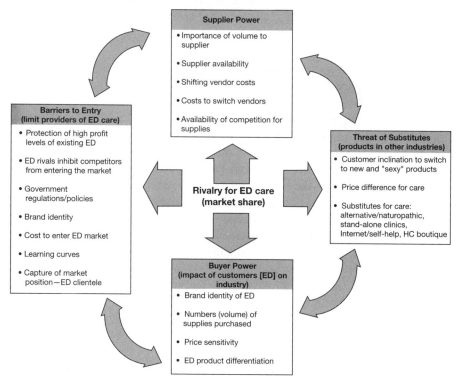

Michael Porter's generic strategies is a third business theory that offers nurses guidance and understanding of business. Thus far, we have looked at the Balanced Scorecard as a means to understanding all the players and content in SP. Then we looked at how the Five Forces define the components in the strategic review. The generic strategies[5] further define advantage. Advantage is cost leadership (low cost, high volume, do more for less); differentiation (offer a unique product—the "only" regional Level I trauma center); and focus strategy (be the best at, or "known" for, something specific—"the" heart hospital).

These are common business theories that nurses may encounter. There are many business theorists, but we chose to highlight Kaplan, Norton, and Porter because as of this writing, they are the contemporary leaders in strategic

---

[5]"Generic" because they are applicable to any industry or enterprise

planning management. Although they have revolutionized the way business is conducted, it is important to note that they are a very small sample of the multitude of drivers in this diverse field. If you would like to dig deeper, in Appendix 8, we have included a bibliography[6] of some of the best and brightest leaders and theorists of strategy.

STRATEGIC PLANNING LOOKS A LOT LIKE THE NURSING PROCESS!

Let's begin with a quick review of the nursing process. So, there are the infamous care plans, not necessarily critical thinking. There are critical paths that resemble checklists, again not really critical thinking. However, when initiated, a care plan or critical path should engage critical thinking regarding the patient's condition and progress based on the science and art of care. Taylor, Lillis, and LeMone (2005) defined the nursing process as "a systematic method that directs . . . [provides] assessment, . . . [utilizes the] nursing diagnosis, . . . [defines expected] outcomes of care, . . . implement[s] care, . . . and evaluate[s] results" (p. 199). If nurses functioned as automatons, this recipe for care would not involve the dynamics of human interaction and the tenets of problem-solving.[7]

The five steps of the nursing process require the application of critical thinking. In their book, *Teaching IOM Implications of the Institute of Medicine Reports for Nursing Education*, Finkelman and Kenner defined critical thinking as having five steps (see Table 8-6) that allow one to rationally consider solutions to a problem.

Nursing care is not conducted in a vacuum. We engage in lifelong learning, curiosity, questioning, open-mindedness, abstraction, and reasoning with clients, peers, and students for a living. In a variety of settings and cultural contexts and among complex sociopolitical factors, nurses methodically solve problems every day. Administrators work in complex environments on a daily basis and, like nurses, methodically solve problems every day.

The predominant role of nursing is evidence-based care derived from assessment. Put succinctly, strategic planning is evidence-based actions derived from assessment. Excellence in care is a direct result of applied critical thinking. Successful strategic thinking and the SP process are the direct results of applied critical thinking.

Business models/theories and nursing models/theories are not far apart. The Institute of Medicine (IOM) has created a business-based healthcare blueprint. The IOM is "at the center of the current restructuring of healthcare

---

[6]Please see the *Harvard Business Review*, January 2008; http://hbr.harvardbusiness.org.
[7]The nursing process is (1) assess, (2) diagnose, (3) plan, (4) implement, and (5) evaluate.

Table 8-6   Finkelman and Kenner's Five Steps of Critical Thinking

1. Adopt the attitude of a critical thinker (attitude of inquiry)
2. Recognize and avoid critical thinking hindrances (consider barriers to the problem)
3. Identify and characterize arguments (identify possible causes and their etiology)
4. Evaluate information sources (reliability and thoroughness)
5. Evaluate arguments (look at all angles)

Source: Finkelman & Kenner, 2007, pp. 66–67.

delivery systems and the movement toward interprofessional work" (Finkelman & Kenner, 2007, p. xi). There is a national trend in generic business practice and in healthcare business toward metaleadership and interdisciplinary care, and away from the silos that we have communicated from for centuries. It can no longer be about "nursing models and theories," "medical models and theories," and "business models and theories." The chasms in care require an integration of professions of care, and nurses are the architects of empowered care reform.

IMAGINEERING AND BRAINSTORMING: BRINGING IT TOGETHER

We have condensed a great deal of theory in this chapter. We would like to give you an opportunity to apply the principles of strategic planning theory. We have used the example of an ED throughout this chapter to demonstrate the use of the Balanced Scorecard and the Five Forces. For real change in the profession of nursing, all nurses will need to claim their voice in the architectural redesign of care. The following two templates (Figures 8-6 and 8-7) are for you to try your hand at imagineering (defined by Walt Disney as master planning, creative development, design, engineering, production, project management, and research and development) care. Imagineering has become a common term for brainstorming and strategic vision at its finest. For this exercise, choose a work setting that is relevant to you. If you could make your setting the best, what variables would need to be included? Every employee has ideas for improving his or her workplace. Now is your chance! What can you imagineer for nursing? Be the architect of change and create a Balanced Scorecard and Five Forces diagram. Who knows, you might share it with the next strategic planning team at your organization!

Theory can be intimidating, but unveiled, it explains why we do what we do. It is the foundation that allows us to critically think in order to address a myriad of issues, including improving work conditions, profits, patient outcomes,

Figure 8-6   Design your Balanced Scorecard.

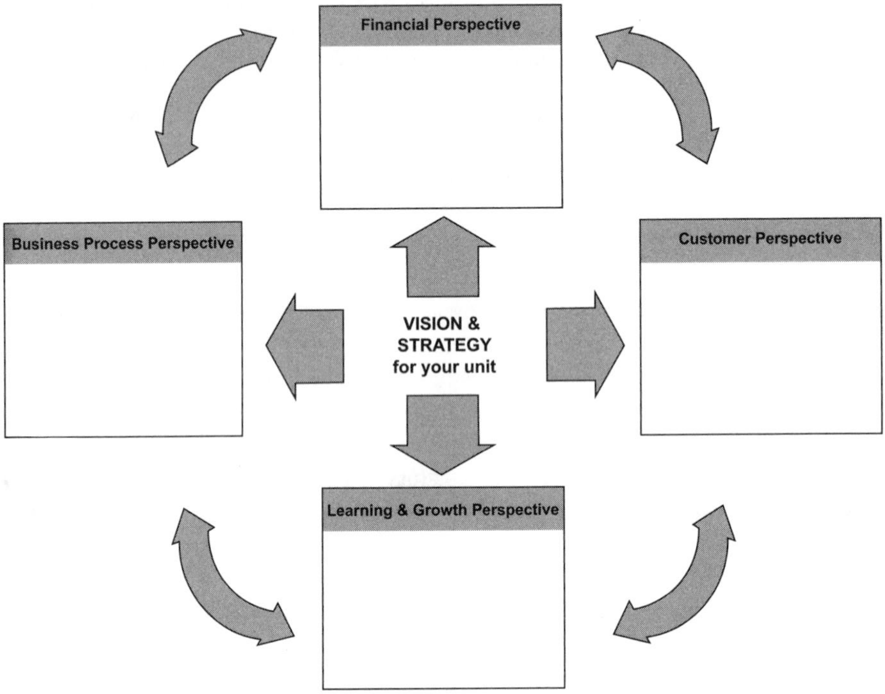

and employee retention; decreasing error rates and employee injuries; and developing collaborative partnerships.

The IOM is asking that we break down silos in order to create bridges to cross the cascade of quality chasms. Aligning theories of business and care is pivotal to constructing the problem-solving partnerships that will empower nursing. In the paper, "Meta-Leadership and National Emergency Preparedness Strategies to Build Government Connectivity," the authors describe the ill effects of traditional discipline-specific silos: "Suffice it to say that the silo effect of distinct cultures, budgets, and narrowly focused career ascendancy compels (government) agencies toward self-protectiveness, insularity, and allegiance to their own agency-based advocacy and independence" (Marcus, Dorn, & Henderson, 2007, p. 1). "Meta-leaders are those who encourage people and organizations to extend beyond their traditional scope of interest and activity" (p. 7). Imagine where this can take nursing.

Figure 8-7   Design your Five Forces.

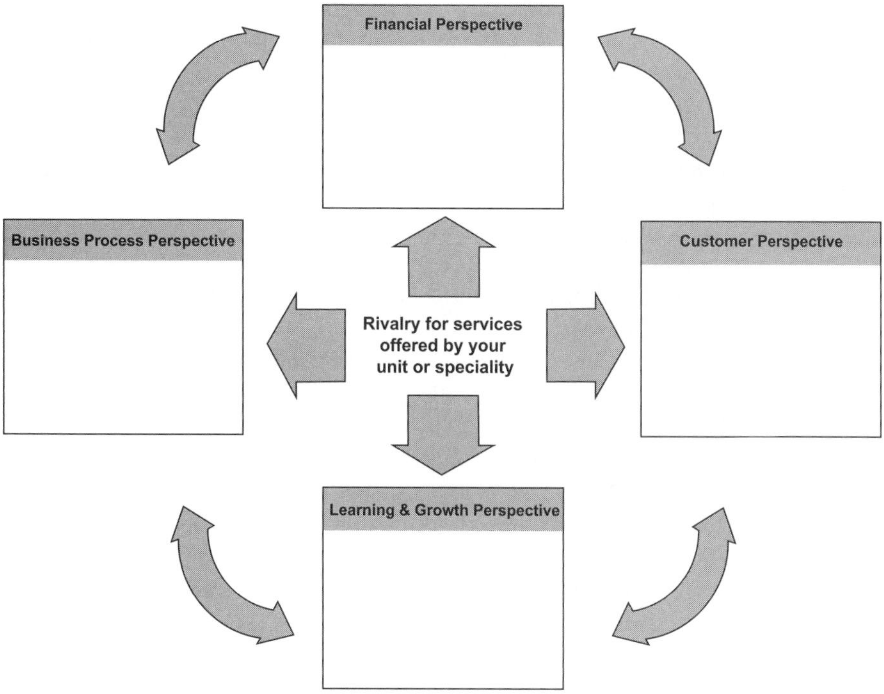

REVIEW QUESTIONS

1. What are the three crucial roles in SP?
2. Define the purpose of a theory.
3. How do values and vision impact the role of the strategic architect?
4. Using an affinity diagram, what similarities exist between nursing and business theory?
5. Employing Porter's Five Forces, diagram how President Washington's health care was decided in the last days of his life.

REFERENCES

Aiken, L., Clarke, S., Sloane, D., Sochalski, J., & Silber, J. (2002). Hospital nurse staffing and patient mortality, nurse burnout, and job dissatisfaction. *Journal of the American Medical Association, 288*(16), 1987–1993.

EmaxHealth. (2008). *Complications after cardiac surgery increase hospital costs.* Retrieved December 27, 2008, from http://emaxhealth.com/80/23141.html

Finkelman, A., & Kenner, C. (2007). *Teaching IOM implications of the Institute of Medicine Reports for Nursing Education.* Silver Spring, MD: American Nurses Association.

Kaplan, R., & Norton, D. (1996). *The Balanced Scorecard: Translating strategy into action.* Boston: Harvard Business School Press.

Kaplan, R., & Norton, D. (2008). Mastering the management system. *Harvard Business Review, 86*(1), 63–77.

Lagente, V., Planquois, J. M., Leclerc, O., Schmidlin, F., & Bertrand, C. (2007). Oxidative stress is an important component of airway inflammation in mice exposed to cigarette smoke or lipopolysaccharide. *Clinical and Experimental Pharmacology and Physiology, 35*(5–6), 601–605.

Marcus, L., Dorn, B., & Henderson, J. (2007). *Meta-leadership and national emergency preparedness.* Retrieved December 27, 2008, from http://209.9.235.208/CMSuploads/Meta-Leadership-(3)-38488.pdf

Porter, M. (2008). The five competitive forces that shape strategy. *Harvard Business Review, 86*(1), 79–93.

Seigworth, G. (2002). *A brief history of bloodletting.* Retrieved December 23, 2008, from http://www.pbs.org/wnet/redgold/printable/p_bloodlettinghistory.html

Tatum, LLC. (2008). *Industries: Healthcare.* Retrieved December 28, 2008, from http://www.tatumllc.com/industries/healthcare.asp

Taylor, C., Lillis, C., & LeMone, P., (2005). *Fundamentals of nursing: The art and science of nursing care* (5th ed.). Philadelphia: Lippincott Williams & Wilkins.

Vadakan, V. (2002). *The asphyxiating and exanguinating death of President George Washington.* Retrieved December 23, 2008, from http://xnet.kp.org/permanentjournal/spring04/time.html

APPENDIX 8

Bibliography

Management System Tool Kit—From the *Harvard Business Review*, January 2008, in the article "Mastering the Management System" by Kaplan and Norton (see http://hbr.harvardbusiness.org/)

DEVELOP STRATEGY

Competitive Strategy

Michael E. Porter, *Competitive Advantage: Creating and Sustaining Superior Performance*, Free Press, 1985 (republished with a new introduction, 1998)

Michael E. Porter, *Competitive Strategy: Techniques for Analyzing Industries and Competitors*, Free Press, 1980 (republished with a new introduction, 1998)

Michael E. Porter, "What Is Strategy?" *Harvard Business Review*, November–December 1996

Chris Zook and James Allen, *Profit from the Core: Growth Strategy in an Era of Turbulence*, Harvard Business School Press, 2001

Resource-Based Strategy

Jay B. Barney, *Gaining and Sustaining Competitive Advantage* (3rd edition), Prentice-Hall, 2006

Jay B. Barney and Delwyn N. Clark, *Resource-Based Theory: Creating and Sustaining Competitive Advantage*, Oxford University Press, 2007

David J. Collis and Cynthia A. Montgomery, "Competing on Resources: Strategy in the 1990s," *Harvard Business Review*, July–August 1995

Gary Hamel and C. K. Prahalad, *Competing for the Future*, Harvard Business School Press, 1994

Blue Ocean Strategy

W. Chan Kim and Renée Mauborgne, *Blue Ocean Strategy: How to Create Uncontested Market Space and Make the Competition Irrelevant*, Harvard Business School Press, 2005

Disruptive Strategy

Clayton M. Christensen and Michael E. Raynor, *The Innovator's Solution: Creating and Sustaining Successful Growth*, Harvard Business School Press, 2003

Emergent Strategy

Gary Hamel, "Strategy Innovation and the Quest for Value," *Sloan Management Review*, Winter 1998

Henry Mintzberg, "Crafting Strategy," *Harvard Business Review*, July–August 1987

Translate the Strategy

Robert S. Kaplan and David P. Norton, *The Strategy-Focused Organization: How Balanced Scorecard Companies Thrive in the New Business Environment*, Harvard Business School Press, 2000

Robert S. Kaplan and David P. Norton, *Strategy Maps: Converting Intangible Assets into Tangible Outcomes*, Harvard Business School Press, 2004

Robert S. Kaplan and David P. Norton, *The Execution Premium: Linking Strategy to Operations for Competitive Advantage*, Harvard Business School Press, 2008

PLAN OPERATIONS

Process Improvement

Wayne W. Eckerson, *Performance Dashboards: Measuring, Monitoring, and Managing Your Business*, John Wiley & Sons, 2006

Michael Hammer, *Beyond Reengineering: How the Process-Centered Organization Is Changing Our Work and Our Lives*, HarperBusiness, 1996

Peter S. Pande, Robert P. Neuman, and Roland R. Cavanagh, *The Six Sigma Way: How GE, Motorola, and Other Top Companies Are Honing Their Performance*, McGraw-Hill, 2000

James P. Womack, Daniel T. Jones, and Daniel Roos, *The Machine That Changed the World: The Story of Lean Production*, Macmillan, 1990

Budgeting and Planning Resource Capacity

Jeremy Hope and Robin Fraser, *Beyond Budgeting: How Managers Can Break Free from the Annual Performance Trap*, Harvard Business School Press, 2003

Robert S. Kaplan and Steven R. Anderson, *Time-Driven Activity-Based Costing: A Simpler and More Powerful Path to Higher Profits*, Harvard Business School Press, 2007

TEST AND ADAPT STRATEGY

Dennis Campbell, Srikant Datar, Susan L. Kulp, and V. G. Narayanan, *Testing Strategy Formulation and Implementation Using Strategically Linked Performance Measures*, HBS Working Paper, 2006

Thomas H. Davenport and Jeanne G. Harris, *Competing on Analytics: The New Science of Winning*, Harvard Business School Press, 2007

Anthony J. Rucci, Steven P. Kirn, and Richard T. Quinn, "The Employee-Customer-Profit Chain at Sears," *Harvard Business Review*, January–February 1998

This bibliography of the *Management System Tool Kit* was retrieved 12/28/2008 from: http://hbr.harvardbusiness.org/2008/01/mastering-the-management-system/ar/1

CHAPTER 9

Understanding Change Theory: Strategic Planning Change Agents

OBJECTIVES

1. Define change.
2. Explain the impact of a paradigm shift.
3. Identify motivators of change.
4. Compare management and leadership.
5. Describe Lewin's three stages of change.
6. Review Prochaska and DiClemente's five stages of change.
7. List common barriers to change.

The change process is a universal constant in nursing. This chapter examines this change process and agents. It asks the reader to consider examples of change as a component of best practice, and the role of change agents. The chapter concludes with an opportunity for readers to assess their "change quotient" and identify their personal barriers to change.

ORCHESTRATING CHANGE AROUND A CHANGELESS CORE

What good would a strategic plan be if met with resistance? The change agent helps people and systems shift the gears that are necessary to implement a strategic plan. In the book *The Heart of Change: Real-Life Stories of How People Change Their Organizations*, Kotter and Cohen (2007) stated that change must be transformational in order to succeed in today's increasingly turbulent world. Through this text, we have built a case for transformational change within nursing. The nursing crisis creates an imperative for professional renewal. Imagine if each nurse led a change within his or her immediate

Figure 9-1   Role of the change agent in the SP process.

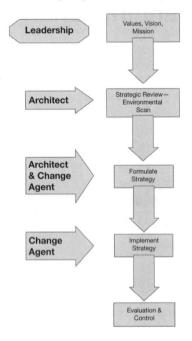

work environment and continued to share that experience with peers in the community.

Nursing understands change. Nurses have studied the concepts that alter health behaviors of individuals and communities. A change agent is the second key role in the strategic planning (SP) process (Kaplan & Norton, 1996). Figure 9-1 identifies the role of the change agent in the SP process.

Dr. Stephen R. Covey[1] (2004) described today's business environment as permanent white water. Change as a constant requires a changeless core based on well-defined and universally understood principles. The nursing profession is an integral part of a change process in the business of health care, which has swung like a giant pendulum over the past few decades. The factors that have impacted the ongoing changes have challenged nursing's core principles— stresses that exposed weaknesses in the paradigm and culture of care.

---

[1]Author of *The 8th Habit: From Effectiveness to Greatness.*

PARADIGMS IN NURSING

A paradigm is a model or pattern of thinking, doing, and being. A paradigm change is commonly referred to as a "paradigm shift." Box 9-1 describes an example of a paradigm shift that occurred in one of our classrooms.

Nursing has undergone many significant paradigm shifts in the past 150 years. In 1854, nursing practice changed forever when Florence Nightingale and 38 other nurses were sent to Scutari, Turkey, to aid physicians in the Crimean War. The doctors saw no need for nurses and did not want them there. Although unwelcome, Ms. Nightingale applied her knowledge and vision of sanitation processes to the dire circumstances. After 154 years, we continue to refer to the impact she had on care. Under her care, the mortality rate dropped from 60% to 2% (American Association of the History of Nursing, Inc., 2008). Applying mathematical principles and statistics (a strategic review), she not only changed the practice of nurses, but she also gave the profession creditability, leading the way to a respectable profession for women.

Using the above example of the student and Florence Nightingale, what caused the paradigm shifts? In neither instance was the shift easy or comfortable. Significant change is often fraught with resistance, chaos, and discomfort.

Box 9-1 Paradigm Shift

A learner came to class late and was disruptive, argumentative, and rude to other learners. She openly professed disdain for people of ethnic or racial backgrounds that were different from her own, and she refused to interact with any of her fellow learners in or outside of class. She had few friends, received poor grades, and was isolated in the classroom, but she was able to meet the requirements necessary to advance to the second semester. The second semester, that same student offered to do a presentation describing her travels to a resource-poor country. What unfolded was our meeting a young woman who had been gang-raped at gunpoint by men of a racial background different from hers; she was now fighting herpes and the fear of developing AIDS, not to mention the tremendous psychological and emotional ravages of such a tragically violent act. She had not intended to discuss any of that in her presentation, but the wounds were so intense that her story needed to be told (from that point on, her grades, friendships, and student nursing career blossomed). Do you see how your view, your paradigm, of this learner completely changed—shifted? Ours certainly did; our lives were enriched by this brave, intelligent, and deeply compassionate young woman who, as it turned out, did not have any deep prejudices and became a skilled and competent nurse. She also returned to the same country to volunteer her skills as a nurse—to help the very culture where she had been so deeply harmed. A tremendous personal paradigm shift!

Although change does not *require* pain, pain can be a strong motivator. Real change starts with a motivator or a team of motivators. That nursing is in crisis is our painful motivator.

> As hospitals' reimbursements, revenues, and margins have been squeezed by private and government payers, patient-to-nurse ratios have increased, nursing salaries have fallen behind other sectors, overtime has increased, and job satisfaction has plummeted . . . stress, irregular working hours, declining working conditions, low morale, and frustration at providing suboptimal care have amplified the shortage as disaffected nurses leave their jobs. (Institute for the Future, 2003, p. 104)

Nursing is ripe with motivators and poised for dramatic shifts in paradigm. Figure 9-2 awakens the memories of why challenges are often necessary for positive change.

Nursing has a rich history of care, and every major advance required a break from traditional thinking and practice. Significant change evolves from shifts in paradigm. Shifts occur as a natural outflow of education, inquiry, positive beliefs in nursing's ability to make a difference, and dedication to excellence. Has pain become a chief motivator for change in care? Nursing must choose motivating drivers, lest it continue on the path of pain—of crisis. Ask any patient; focus on pain leads to more pain.

STRATEGIC REVIEW: NURSING'S DIVERSITY

There are many examples for change in nursing. We will use one example throughout this chapter to discuss change and change theory. First, let's conduct a mini–strategic review on one component of the nursing profession: our demographic.

The Nursing Demographic: A Need for Diversity

Nursing has made great strides and responsibly solved phenomenal challenges since the 1872 inception of the profession at the New England Hospital for Women and Children, the home of the first professional nurse training program in the United States.[2] Linda Richards was the first to graduate in October 1873 after a 12-month training program. The first professionally trained African

---

[2] American Association of the History of Nursing; aahn.org.

Figure 9-2   Care is timeless, yet evolutionary.

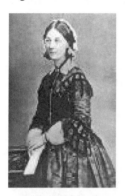 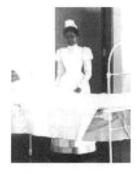 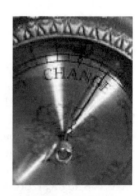

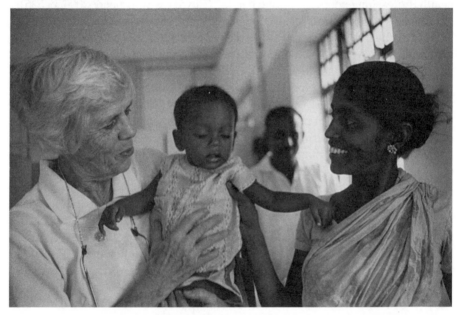

Florence Nightingale circa 1860; African American nurse circa 1880; barometer for change; and Lillian Carter, nurse, Peace Corps volunteer, and namesake of The Lillian Carter Center for International Nursing, Emory University, Atlanta, GA.

Lillian Carter photo courtesy of Peace Corps.

American nurse was Mary Eliza Mahoney, who graduated in 1879. Even though one of our first professional nurses was of African American descent, today only 21% of RNs are minorities (Bureau of Labor Statistics [BLS], 2008). Despite the fact that 34% of the United States is comprised of minorities (U.S. Census Bureau, 2008), "some U.S. racial and ethnic minorities continue to be grossly underrepresented among health professionals, despite the increasing diversity of the U.S. population" (Institute of Medicine [IOM], 2004).[3]

"The number of African American, Hispanic American, Asian American, Hawaiian Native/Pacific Islander, and Native American/Alaskan Native students enrolled in nursing programs is significantly lower than the percent of the population they comprise; generally, they are considered to be the underrepresented groups in nursing schools" (AllNursingSchools.com, 2008). "Nursing schools have the highest proportion of underrepresented minority students of any health profession except for public health" (Cowen & Moorhead, 2006, p. 535).

Many schools of nursing have amended their curricula to include concepts of cultural diversity, yet 79% of the profession comprises members of the dominant culture.[4] "Women from underrepresented groups have been relegated primarily to roles of servitude within the healthcare system as nursing aides or as practical nurses . . . [this] has limited severely the ability to advance within the mainstream of nursing" (Cowen et al., 2006, p. 532). "Since the 1960s, considerable advances have been made in the ability of women in previously underrepresented groups to participate in all levels of society. But in nursing the situation has remained static, with little advancement on the part of nurses of color" (Cowen et al., 2006, p. 532).

Debating the many reasons and justifications for these data is a gargantuan undertaking; what is relevant for our strategic review is to ask the question, Can't any nurse care for any client? The answer is no. In its 2002 report, the IOM found that communication barriers between minority clientele and nurses had negative effects on patient outcomes and quality indicators (BLS, 2008). The BLS also stated, "Studies suggest that the healthcare needs of patients from minority groups are not always being met" (Lien & BLS, 2004). The *National Healthcare Disparity Report* (Agency for Healthcare Research and Quality [AHRQ], 2003) stated that "the evidence of the damaging health consequences of racial and ethnic disparities in health care continues to be overwhelming." "Barbee and Gibson (2001) state that a culture of racism exists in nursing education" (Cowen et al., 2006, p. 547).

---

[3]See http://www.iom.edu/CMS/3740/4888.aspx to learn more about the text from the IOM *In the Nation's Compelling Interest: Ensuring Diversity in the Health Care Workforce.*
[4]White or Caucasian.

Disparity in the profession's demographics mirrors the disparity in care; nursing needs to address and create strategies to correct this chasm. We'll use disparity in the nursing demographic as a basis for strategic management of care throughout our discussion of change and change theory, with strategic planning as a crucial tool and change management as the tool that facilitates strategic thinking and implementation. The architect designs the strategies; the change agent enables a shifting paradigm within which the strategic plan might be brought to fruition.

Considering the demographic disparity in nursing, which paradigm(s) must shift in order to culturally align the profession of care with the population served? Please list, in order, how you will prioritize your ideas for necessary changes (paradigm shifts):

1._____

2._____

3._____

4._____

(Please send your ideas to Michele@nursesfornursesinternational.com or Leann@nursesfornursesinternational.com; we will post your ideas on our Web site. Or, better yet, submit an article to a nursing journal!)

IF "CHANGE IS THE ONLY CONSTANT," WHY IS IT SO HARD? CHANGE MANAGEMENT AND CHANGE THEORY

Try as we may to stick with the status quo, change is omnipresent. As we begin this section, please take a look at Table 9-1, Four Key Elements to Anticipating Change. Before we can embark on understanding the course of change, we must first recognize that we naturally go through stages of an assessment. Think about these four tasks as you read this section on change management.

Table 9-1   Four Key Elements to Anticipating Change

1. Identifying prevailing paradigm(s)
2. Recognizing a need (for change)
3. Assessing the tenets of the situation (strategic review)
4. Identifying which paradigm(s) must shift in order to effect change

We have all heard that "change is the only constant." Yet, people tend to resist change. Why this dichotomy? Stop for a moment and write down the feelings and thoughts that come to mind when you hear the word *change*. You may be surprised at the wide range of emotions the exercise elicits.

Leaders must be able to "deconstruct the culture to change outcomes" (Freshwater, Taylor, & Sherwood, 2008, p. 139). It is a relatively simple task to enforce some changes. Switching to a needless system can be accomplished by changing vendors, stocking supplies, and educating staff. There might be some grumbling, but nurses will shift their practice, even without significant buy-in. This autocratic approach to change is where the precept of management dogma resides. Leadership pilots individuals and organizations toward excellence (recall the management of the industry worker versus the leading of knowledge workers).

Referring to our demographic example, it is possible to force the issue of diversity as well. In 1957, the Little Rock Nine[5] were enrolled at Central High School in Little Rock, Arkansas, resulting in the Little Rock Crisis.[6] This was a decisive showdown in the civil rights movement, which led to the long overdue transformation in national consciousness—a consciousness that continues to evolve and mature. How would you categorize the desegregation efforts in the 1950s and into the 1960s? Were these leadership efforts, management efforts, or both? Were there any other ways to shift our national paradigm regarding segregation?

How then should we address the chasm in diversity that plagues nursing education and the profession? The Little Rock Crisis forced a shift in our national culture—our national paradigm. Ask yourself the question again: Was that leadership, or was it management? Which does nursing need? Is one necessary for the other? Are they exclusive or dependent?

But is it always a leader who instigates significant change? Dr. Stephen R. Covey, an expert on leadership and organizations for more than 40 years, asserts that change is a result of an individual or group whose members are able to use their true nature and gifts to create a vision, to find their voice to express that vision, and to inspire others to find their voice (Covey, 2004). Victor Frankl[7] (1984) wrote this about change: "What man actually needs is not

---

[5]Nine African American students chosen by the National Association for the Advancement of Colored People (NAACP) to be the first black students to enter an all-White high school.
[6]The Arkansas governor, using National Guard troops, blocked the nine students' entry to the school. President Eisenhower facilitated a court injunction to let the students attend; the students then came under the protection of the army for the ensuing tense school year.
[7]Victor Frankl (1905–1997) was an Austrian psychiatrist whose writings include *Man's Search for Meaning*.

a tensionless state but rather the striving and struggling for some goal worthy of him. What he needs is not the discharge of tension at any cost, but the call of a potential meaning waiting to be fulfilled by him" (p. 166). Stretching back across time, it seems that change is not the domain of leaders or power; it is as Covey and Frankl attested: It is about a clear purpose. In 1882, T. L. Haines and L. W. Yaggy wrote that "will is the root; knowledge the stems and leaves; feeling the flower . . . He who resolves on doing a thing, by that very resolution scales the barriers to it, and secures its achievement" (Haines & Yaggy, 1882, p. 217).

So how do nurse change agents change things? Is it a simple matter of determination, a clear vision and set of strategies? There is the ever-popular ritual of New Year's resolutions and the spike in the gym memberships and fitness gear sales. How does that work? Have you ever started a new position filled with great ideas, only to unwittingly leave a path of antagonism in the wake of your well-intentioned efforts? Being in charge of change—as a change agent—can be a slippery slope of successive disasters. Change does not have to be painful, and if change is to be sustainable, it must flow from respect for all involved and affected. We need not go it alone; change theories help to navigate and facilitate paradigm shifts and effect positive change by giving us tools and methods that have been validated through research.

Kurt Lewin, the generally accepted founder of organizational psychology, advanced his three-stage theory on organizational change in the 1940s (Figure 9-3). He also coined the term *force-field analysis*, which has taken on broader meanings in current management theories. In 1994, Prochaska and DiClemente created the Transtheoretical Model (TTM) of change (as change relates to altering health behaviors), which has found that people move through five stages in the implementation of healthy practices or the cessation of poor health choices (see Table 9-2). Lippitt, Watson, and Westley (1958) added to Lewin's three-stage theory to create seven steps that are directed to the role and responsibilities of the change agent (see Figure 9-4). First, we offer an overview of each of their theories; we then

Figure 9-3 Lewin's three stages of change.

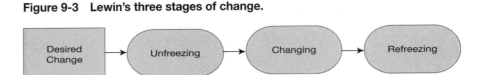

Table 9-2   Prochaska and DiClemente's Five Stages of Change Model

Stage of Change	Characteristics	Behaviors
Pre-contemplation	Not considering change; either unaware or undereducated	Ignorance as bliss or avoidance
Contemplation	"Sitting on the fence" stage—not considering change within a month	Ambivalent; aware but not impressed by any need to change
Preparation	Some experience with change—planning to act within 1 month	Increased awareness; recognizes a need for change
Action	Implements change as incremental; practicing new behavior 3–6 months	Changed social cues; changed support systems; self-esteem for self-efficacy
Maintenance	6 months to 5 years; continued commitment	Rewards system; coping mechanisms

Figure 9-4   Lippitt, Watson, and Westley's steps and roles for the change agent.

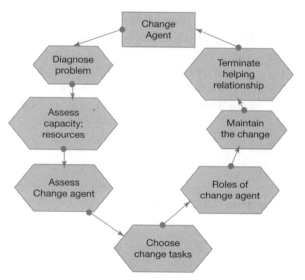

apply them to our nursing demographic dilemma in a unique way (see Figure 9-5).

Lewin's Three Stages of Change

Lewin identified three stages—unfreezing, change, and refreezing—to categorize the complex human processes, attitudes, and thoughts that affect a change process. In the unfreezing stage, the change subject(s) is in a pattern of habits that offers a sense of dependability and security; Lewin called this

Figure 9-5 Change theories of Lewin; Prochaska and DiClemente; and Lippitt, Watson, and Westley redesigned to address strategic initiatives in nursing.

Strategic Plan	Lewin's Three Stages		
	Unfreezing	Change	Refreezing
Strategic review; factors related to challenges in nursing PDC 1–2 and L 1–3	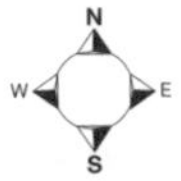		
Driving Forces PDC 3 and L 2–3	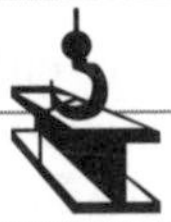		
Restraining Forces PDC 3 and L 2–3			
Formulate strategy and set tasks PDC 4 and L 4		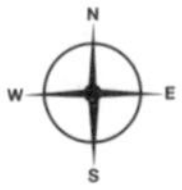	
Implement strategy/change PDC 4 and L 4–5		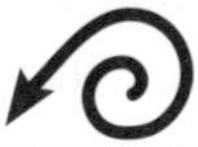	
Evaluate strategy/change PDC 5 and L 5–6			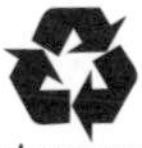
Culturalize strategy/change PDC 5 and L 7			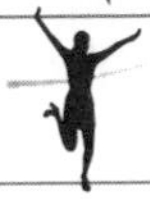
PDC = Prochaska & DiClemente, L = Lippitt et al.			

Source: Sare, 2008.

quasi-stationary equilibria.[8] The task of this stage is to use force-field analysis to assess which forces contribute to the status quo. The next step to unfreezing is to determine which of these forces are positive (driving) and which are restraining (negative). Finally, the unfreezing stage determines which forces need to increase and/or which forces need to decrease in order to achieve the desired change results. The overarching task of unfreezing is to release old patterns.

The second stage is change (or "moving to a new level"). Within this stage, the change subject(s) adapts the forces—patterns, attitudes, beliefs, practices, thoughts—that facilitate the identified change. The goal of this stage is to be working within the change; change is occurring that actualizes the goal(s) of change.

The third stage, refreezing, establishes the new patterns, practices, beliefs, attitudes, and thoughts as the norm; they have become a habit that replaces old ways of being. This is the stage at which a new modus operandi is culturalized. Refreezing seeks to prevent backsliding, or a return to the old patterns. The theory of these three stages is complex, but understand that skipping over any one of the three renders change ineffective or unsustainable. Always, change is dynamic.

Prochaska and DiClemente's Five Stages of Change

Nurses may be very familiar with the change process of Prochaska and DiClemente. All nurses, at every level, are charged with the responsibility of patient education. From teaching insulin administration to showing a patient how to manage a Jackson-Pratt wound vac, nurses teach. The purpose of teaching is to effect positive change; teaching is a strategy to implement change. The Five Stages of Change model identifies common human change behavior and offers some guidelines as to how and when a patient will adopt new patterns (habits), beliefs, feelings, and thoughts. Teaching falls on deaf ears if the learner is not ready to listen. Table 9-3 lists other concepts to consider that are associated with readiness to learn.

Lippitt, Watson, and Westley Stages (and Roles) for the Change Agent

Lippitt (a colleague of Lewin's), Watson, and Westley added to the three stages. They addressed the need for understanding how a change agent works with

---

[8]Kurt Lewin, 1957, Massachusetts Institute of Technology.

Table 9-3   Additional Considerations for Change Readiness

- Emotional state—grief, fear, body image, anxiety
- Pain or discomfort—ability to attend to the teaching
- Age, culture, gender
- Language, literacy, learning style
- Medications, nutrition, physiologic condition
- Mental health

---

and within the change process. The strategic planning liaison is similar to a change agent and may fill the same role. The first task is to diagnose the problem (strategic review). As a continuation of the environmental scan, the change agent then determines (second stage) the level of motivation of individuals, units, or systems. This stage also assesses the capacity for change (e.g., we want to add 5000 new minority student nurses, but are there sufficient schools of nursing to do so?). The third stage is to assess the change agents themselves; do they have stamina, personality traits conducive to interpersonal success, authority or necessary power, etc.? The fourth stage is similar to the strategic planning phase—formulate strategies, those tasks that will lead to goal completion. The fifth stage communicates the roles and responsibilities of the change agent to all stakeholders. The sixth stage is similar to the refreezing; this is the "maintain the change" stage. The seventh stage withdraws the change agent from its roles and responsibilities; the change agent's job is complete when the change is part of the culture.

- Stages 1–3—aligned with the unfreezing stage
- Stages 4–5—aligned with the change or moving to a new stage
- Stages 6–7—aligned with the refreezing stage

The strategic planning process will lead to a dead end if the principles guiding change are neglected. Here we offered the basis for three leading change theories. Now let's apply these theories to our demographic diversity dilemma in a unique way that combines these theories. Change is a complex process, and nursing is a complex profession that is multidimensional and dynamic. A multidimensional approach is necessary to address the disparity in nursing's demographic (Exhibit 9-1).

Exhibit 9-1   Change Theory Applied Through the Strategic Planning Process

I.   Strategic review:
  A. Unfreezing (in Figure 9-6, the compass represents the need to determine or align with direction—values and mission)
    1. Lippitt et al.—Stage I—diagnosis. Cultural disparity in nursing (see justification in paragraphs 2–5 in the subsection titled Strategic Review: Nursing's Diversity).
    2. Lippitt et al.—Stage II—assess the motivation and capacity for change (external and internal force fields; chasms in care related to cultural incongruences—disparity, access, errors, costs, quality of life, morbidity, mortality, life expectancy by race, disease rates by demographics, for example, AIDS, diabetes, heart disease). The core of nursing is care; for this example, we are assuming that all nurses and nurse educators are motivated to ensure cultural congruence and competency.
    3. Lippitt et al.—Stage III—assessment of the change agents. Change agents in nursing historically have been theorists, nurse administrators, and nursing organizations. There is only one nurse theorist whose work focuses on cultural competency: Madeline Leininger. Her work does not specifically address the need for more minority nurses, but she espouses the need for a culturally competent healthcare workforce. The 2002 *Nursing's Agenda for the Future: A Call to the Nation* article (ANA) stated that "nursing mirrors the diverse population it serves"; this is incongruent with the stated data from AHRQ and the IOM (as above). In this report, 10 domains of concern requiring action were identified; the 10th domain is diversity (ANA, 2002)—"Vision. . . . Nursing increasingly reflects the population it serves. . . . Primary Strategy [is to] create diversity and cultural competence through educational programs and standards in the workplace. Increase diversity of faculty, students and curricula in all academic and continuing education"[1] (ANA, 2002): Nursing change agents are motivated and have the power to effect this change in nursing's demographic.
    4. Prochaska and DiClemente—Stage I—pre-contemplation. National nursing organizations have contemplated the need for diversity. Has the regional, state, community, organization, and individual nurse considered this change? Some top-down government and nongovernment (such as The Joint Commission) regulations have either required or rewarded diversity through grants, scholarships, and fair labor laws. An informal scan reveals that the professional whole of nursing is still in the stage of not considering this change.
    5. Prochaska and DiClemente—Stage II—contemplation. Some pockets of the nursing profession are aware of the chasm in nursing's demographic diversity.
    6. Driving forces[2]: costs, quality, errors, vision, purpose/mission of care, Department of Public Health and Human Services (DPHHS), IOM, The Joint Commission, Centers for Medicare and Medicaid (CMS), AHRQ, etc.
    7. Restraining forces[2]: cost to implement; educational barriers; underrepresentation of minority role models; cultural chasms in education models; history of nursing as a predominantly female Caucasian occupation; largest number of minorities entering the profession through associate's degree programs (the cultural chasm

Exhibit 9-1   *(Continued)*

is greatest at the AP and doctoral levels; Cowen et al., 2006); nurse's image; more career options; difficulty recruiting new nurses; restrained career development options; etc.

II. Formulate Strategy (in Figure 9-6, the compass showing true north represents the formulation of strategy—knowing exactly which direction to take):

A. Change (moving to a new level)

    1. Lippitt et al.—Stage IV—Develop action plan and strategies; DPHHS, IOM, The Joint Commission, CMS, AHRQ, ANA, and the National League for Nursing (NLN). Examples of developed strategies: The NLN mission is to "promote excellence in nursing education to build a strong and diverse nursing workforce . . . and build a diverse membership through comprehensive, inclusive, and aggressive methods" [NLN].[3] The University of California at San Francisco Center for the Health Professions sets staffing ratios as a strategy. The IOM sets three strategies to address healthcare workforce diversity: assess and describe benefits to diversity, assess institutional and policy-level strategies that may increase diversity, and identify mechanisms to garner broad support among health professional leaders (IOM, 2004).

    2. Prochaska and DiClemente—Stage IV—preparation. Some pockets of the nursing profession are aware of the chasm in nursing's demographic diversity and have taken steps to improve diversity and cultural responsiveness (this is aligned with Lippitt et al., Stage IV).

III. Implement Strategy (in Figure 9-6, the circular arrow represents the project's [strategies/change] readiness to move forward):

A. Change continued (moving to a new level)

    1. Lippitt et al.—Stages IV and V—as described previously. Strategies become task oriented, and specific action steps are implemented. At the national level, many of the strategies are being implemented; some remain suggestions, ideas, or unsupported mandates.[4]

    2. Prochaska and DiClemente—Stage IV—as mentioned previously. Strategies become task oriented, and specific action steps are implemented. At the national level, many of the strategies are being implemented; some remain suggestions, ideas, or unsupported mandates.[4]

    3. Prochaska and DiClemente—Stage V—maintenance or continuity. This is closely tied to refreezing, but in Prochaska and DiClemente's definition, this is the stage wherein change is *becoming* culturalized.

IV. Evaluate Strategies/Change Efforts (the process is "recycled" to assess strengths, weaknesses, need for improvement, what to keep, what to discard—hence, it is represented in Figure 9-6 by the recycling symbol):

A. Refreezing

    1. Lippitt et al.—Stage VI—maintain the change. Some change strategies have been implemented, but as of this writing, no significant change has occurred in

(Continued)

Exhibit 9-1   *(Continued)*

nursing's demographics in the past 5 years even though many strategies to improve cultural responsiveness in nursing education have been implemented.

2. Lippitt et al.—Stage VII—gradually terminate the role of the change agent (in this case, their work is far from being done—not there yet).

3. Prochaska and DiClemente—Stage V—maintenance or continuity ongoing—replaced old habits/paradigms. Some change strategies have been implemented, but as of this writing, no significant change has occurred in nursing's demographics in the past 5 years even though many strategies to improve cultural responsiveness in nursing education have been implemented. Their Stage V has not been attained with regard to cultural diversity within nursing.

V. Culturalized Strategy/Change (this cannot be addressed because the problem is not resolved; the happy runner represents project success):
A. Refreezing—unable to proceed—strategies/change unmet.

[1]For a complete copy of this report please go to https://www.ncsbn.org/Plan.pdf.

[2]In Figure 9-5, the beam is a weight that represents restraining forces, and the cable and hook represents driving forces; for change to occur, the driving forces need to exceed or overcome the restraining forces.

[3]To learn more about strategic efforts aimed at diversity at the NLN, please see http://www.nln.org/aboutnln/our mission.htm

[4]Some change strategies have been implemented, but as of this writing, no significant change has occurred in nursing's demographics in the past 5 years even though many strategies to improve cultural responsiveness in nursing education have been implemented.

Figure 9-6 conceptualizes the application of change theory to a nursing challenge being solved through the strategic planning process. We can design the best strategies, but we must be able to get all stakeholders to effectively participate; the strategy must be supported by skillfully applying principles of change. Now, let's give some clarification to Figure 9-6 using the diversity in nursing example.

Recall that the demographic of professional nursing is predominantly Caucasian, but the population whom American nurses serve is at least 30% minorities. The challenge is to create a (strategic) plan to address this chasm. A strategic plan is all about "unfreezing," creating new practices that facilitate some indicator of quality and/or excellence, and then culturalizing, or freezing,

Figure 9-6   Change theory within the strategic planning process simplified.

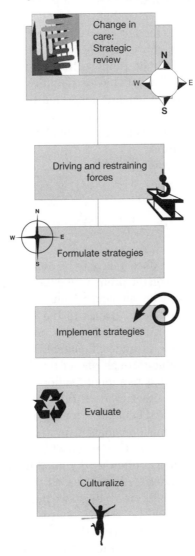

Source: Sare, 2008.

the change. The strategic plan: Improve the cultural responsiveness of nursing. The change: more minority nurses (we are not presuming that this is the only necessary change, but it is a change that we can address here for our example of change theories applied to nursing).

In Exhibit 9-1, we have demonstrated how and where differing change theories are aligned. Lewin did not suppose that three simple stages lead to change. Within his theory, many behavior modification processes facilitate each stage. Prochaska and DiClemente identified five stages of change that likewise have related behavioral tasks. Lippitt et al. expanded Lewin's theory to address change agents, but theirs is closely aligned with the same behavioral principles that he identified.

Figure 9-6 is a symbolic overview of the matrix of change and the strategic planning process.

Barriers to Change

Change is not a bad thing, nor does it have to be difficult. President Obama led a successful campaign based on the premise of change. Change can be empowering, uplifting, and positively life-altering. Change comes about because of an identified need—a motivator. Need comes to the forefront in two ways: by inflicted learning (force, pain or tragedy, etc.) or by self-directed learning (inquiry, expanded worldview, attitudes, facilitated learning, etc.). New information makes change possible through one of two ways: (1) learning that is based on either positive or negative identification, or (2) learning from trial and error (Schein, 2004). In either case, learning causes a new paradigm—a new way of thinking, acting, and being. Learning is one of our best sources for continued motivation; total quality management (TQM), evidence-based practice (EBP), and Magnet Status are all a result of new learning that became a motivator for change. Change is often a very good thing. Change is the only way to shed that pesky scarlet C (change based on sound strategic plans!). Then why are there so many barriers? Why do we need theories? Why don't we do the Nike thing and "just do it"?

As a change agent and one who is both a self-leader and a professional leader, you'll need to know some of the common barriers to change (Table 9-4). These are just a few of the restraining forces that are encountered throughout any change process. Perhaps you can think of others. The take-home lesson is to be aware that whenever you ask a person or system to change, people prefer the status quo—or, as Lewin called it, the "quasi-stationary equilibria." Most people do not want to feel off-balance. They like

Table 9-4 Common Barriers to Change

- Threat of increased workload
- Lack of understanding of the process
- Previous poor experiences with change
- Poor relationships with management
- Lack of leadership
- Ineffective communication across the organization
- Disruption in security—fear of the unknown
- Personalities who prefer linear pragmatism
- Learned conformity
- Mistrust between levels and departments
- Bad strategic planning design
- Fear of failure
- Corporate culture dysfunction
- Victim mentality
- Entrenched habits and culture—threat to identity
- Supposition of inadequacy if individuals do not see the need for change—guilt, threat

knowing what they can and can't do, and they enjoy the rhythm that they create in their job. Change may be seen as upsetting the apple cart; address these barriers early if you want a change or a strategic plan to be successful.

On Being a Culture Change Agent

"There is nothing so powerful as an idea whose time has come."
—Victor Hugo, 1802–1885

Change is not linear, nor is change hierarchical. Change is a process, not a static entity. Change is not a one-time occurrence; change is learning and growth. Change can come from an individual, an aggregate, a community, a team, or an organization. Organizations may employ change agents, but every individual has the power to be the instigator and conductor of change.

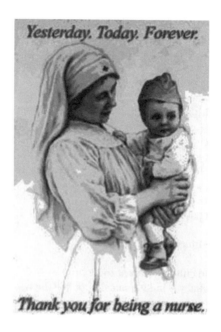

Yesterday. Today. Forever.

Thank you for being a nurse.

Understanding the meaning of, and need for, change, the nurse as an individual and nursing as a profession will be better prepared to be competently proactive and empowered. It is our hope that this text will instigate discussion and facilitate deeper bonds and interlevel respect within the culture of nursing—the culture of care. We nurses have come a long way, but this new century presents us with the opportunity to continually improve on what it means to be a nurse—to be a provider of care.

We have established that change is not easy, but change is absolutely possible and occurs whether or not we want it, whether or not we participate, whether or not we understand, and whether or not we like it. The crisis in our profession happened without much ruckus nationally; change in nursing happened while most nurses kept their heads down and went to work. It was insidious. Nurses can no longer afford to let the tides of change swirl around them; that giant scarlet C has got to go. Thinking about the example of the need to more deeply diversify nursing, what ideas do you have to solve the dilemma? You are a change agent; what do you want to change in nursing, in care?

> *". . . become an island of excellence in a sea of mediocrity . . .*
> *it's contagious."*
> —Dr. Stephen R. Covey, 1932–Present

Before we leave the subject of change, we want to leave you with some ideas about effective change that are outside the traditional academic models but that nonetheless have helped many people actualize their goals. These are ideas and theories that come from the relatively new field of transformational leadership and disciplines that study principles of success. Authors such as Drucker, Blanchard, Kotter, Robbins, Covey, Canfield, Dyer, and many others offer tools and methods for effective change. Please explore the many ways they might help you to be the change that you want to see. We have included a list of these change agents in Appendix 9. We think that you will enjoy further reading on the fascinating area of change—our only constant.

A Little Quiz: Are You Stuck?

1. When was the last time you attended a class on cultural diversity?

   _____

2. What are your concerns about cultural diversity in care? _____

   _____

   _____

3. Describe your experiences with change: _____

   _____

   _____

(Continued)

---

4. Change is: a. good   b. bad   _____

5. Define *cultural competence*: _____

    _____

    _____

6. Change is: a. hard   b. easy   _____

7. I am overworked, underpaid, and underappreciated, and I would not want any more to deal with: T   F

8. I would only agree to a change process or strategic plan if I was paid more: T   F

(We are confident you can interpret the test results yourself.)

REVIEW QUESTIONS

1. What is a paradigm shift?
2. List three examples of "motivators" for change.
3. What are Lewin's three stages of change?
4. Describe Lewin's three stages of change.
5. What are the refreezing stages of Prochaska and DiClemente's five stages of change?
6. What is a barrier to change? List three examples of change barriers.

REFERENCES

Agency for Healthcare Research and Quality (AHRQ). (2003). *National healthcare disparities report 2003: Executive summary.* Retrieved December 20, 2008, from http://www.ahrq.gov/qual/nhdr03/fullreport/exec.htm

AllNursingSchools.com. (2008). *Nursing programs for minorities.* Retrieved April 28, 2009, from http://www.allnursingschools.com/faqs/diversityfaq.php

American Association of the History of Nursing, Inc. (2008). *Marie E. Zakrzewska, 1829–1902.* Retrieved December 30, 2008, from http://www.aahn.org/gravesites/zakrzewska.html

American Nurses Association (ANA). (2002). *Nursing's agenda for the future: A call to action.* Retrieved October 22, 2008, from www.nursingworld.org/MainMenu Categories/HealthcareandPolicyIssues/Reports/AgendafortheFuture.aspx

Bureau of Labor Statistics (BLS). (2008). *Occupational outlook handbook, 2008–09 edition.* Retrieved April 28, 2009, from http://www.bls.gov/oco/ocos083.htm

Covey, S. R. (2004). *The 8th habit: From effectiveness to greatness.* New York: Free Press.

Cowen, P. S., & Moorhead, S. (2006). *Current issues in nursing* (7th ed.). St. Louis, MO: Mosby-Elsevier.

Frankl, V. E. (1984). *Man's search for meaning.* New York: Washington Square Press.

Freshwater, D., Taylor, B. J., & Sherwood, G. (2008). *International textbook of reflective practice in nursing.* West Sussex, UK: Wiley-Blackwell.

Haines, T. L., & Yaggy, L. W. (1882). *The royal path of life.* Chicago: Western Publishing House.

Institute for the Future. (2003). *2003 ten-year forecast* (pp. 1–183). Retrieved May 7, 2009, from http://www.iftf.org/system/files/deliverables/2003_Ten-Year_Forecast.pdf

Institute of Medicine (IOM). (2004). *Institutional and policy-level strategies for increasing the racial and ethnic diversity of the U.S. healthcare workforce.* Retrieved October 10, 2008, from http://www.iom.edu/CMS/3740/4888.aspx

Kaplan, R., & Norton, D. (1996). *The Balanced Scorecard: Translating strategy into action.* Boston: Harvard Business School Press.

Kotter, J. P., & Cohen, D. S. (2002). *The heart of change: Real-life stories of how people change their organizations.* Boston: Harvard Business School Press.

Lien, M., & Bureau of Labor Statistics (BLS). (2004). *Workforce diversity: Opportunities in the melting pot.* Occupational Outlook Quarterly. 28–37. Retrieved December 2, 2008, from http://www.bls.gov/opub/ooq/2004/summer/art02.pdf

National League for Nursing (NLN). (2008). *Mission and goals.* Retrieved October 22, 2008, from http://www.nln.org/aboutnln/ourmission.htm

Schein, E. H. (2004). *Organizational culture and leadership* (3rd ed.). San Francisco: Jossey-Bass.

U.S. Census Bureau. (2008). *U.S. Hispanic population surpasses 45 million: Now 15 percent of total.* Retrieved April 28, 2009, from http://www.census.gov/Press-Release/www/releases/archives/population/011910.html

Change Agents

Ken Blanchard (Author of *The One Minute Manager*)
   The Ken Blanchard Companies
   http://www.kenblanchard.com

Jack Canfield (Author of *The Success Principles*)
   The Jack Canfield Companies
   http://www.jackcanfield.com

Stephen R. Covey (Author of *The 8th Habit: From Effectiveness to Greatness*)
   Franklin Covey Co.
   http://www.franklincovey.com

Peter F. Drucker (Author of *Management Challenges for the 21st Century*)
   The Drucker Institute
   http://www.druckerinstitute.com

Wayne Dyer (Author of *Excuses Begone! How to Change Lifelong Self-Defeating Thinking Habits*)
   http://www.drwaynedyer.com

Napoleon Hill (Author of *Think and Grow Rich*)
   The Napoleon Hill Foundation
   http://www.naphill.org

John P. Kotter (Author of *The Heart of Change: Real-Life Stories of How People Change Their Organizations*)
   http://www.johnkotter.com

Anthony (Tony) Robbins (Author of *Awaken the Giant Within: How to Take Immediate Control of Your Mental, Emotional, Physical and Financial Destiny!*)
   Anthony Robbins Companies
   http://www.tonyrobbins.com/Home/Home.aspx

Mark Victor-Hansen (Author of *The Power of Focus: What the Worlds Greatest Achievers Know about The Secret of Financial Freedom and Success*)
   Mark Victor Hansen & Associates, Inc.
   http://www.markvictorhansen.com/contact.php

CHAPTER 10

Communicating the Strategic Plan

1. Describe examples of nonverbal communication.
2. Explain the components of verbal communication.
3. Review the ANA's communication competencies for nurses.
4. Define metacommunication.
5. Identify the paths of organizational communication.
6. Describe the role of the strategic planning communicator.
7. List barriers to communication.
8. Review de Bono's colored hats analogy.

The third role in strategic planning processes identified by Kaplan and Norton (1996) is the communicator. Positive and effective change cannot be accomplished through poor communication; the best strategic plan (SP) in the world will go nowhere if it is inadequately communicated. At the heart of business, and professional and personal interactions of any kind, lies quality of communication—communication that either drives or restrains, communication that either hinders or helps. The best managers are effective communicators. Good leaders are master communicators. We exist in this world through the many signals, cues, actions, responses, and input that are communicated through all our senses, verbal and nonverbal.

Communication comes in a myriad of forms. There are the verbal and nonverbal techniques that all nurses are familiar with. Verbal techniques encompass what is spoken, signed, or written, and nonverbal comprises body language (which some people are infinitely more skilled at than others) and environmental cues. Communication can occur interpersonally (between people), intrapersonally (self-talk or talk within a discipline), or publicly (to groups). Figure 10-1 demonstrates the role of the communicator in the SP process.

Figure 10-1   Role of the communicator in the SP process.

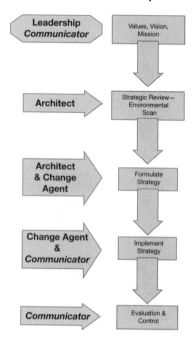

NONVERBAL COMMUNICATION

Have you ever felt misunderstood despite your most articulate efforts? Could it be that your words are usurped by your nonverbal communication? The first nonverbal communicator to consider is the environment or setting. Information conveyed through the environment is a forcible communicator. We set the stage to convey meaning, attitudes, and beliefs; think of a shopping mall and the many storefronts, and the type of customer they attract or repel. Or, think of the different types of healthcare environments and their unique purposes. The decor and layout of a pediatric clinic, a surgical suite, or a chemotherapy unit are designed to impart the particular caring beliefs and technical needs of the clientele—or they should (an ob-gyn whose office was decorated with trophy heads and hunting paraphernalia—not one sign that the primary clientele were women—communicated a strong message about the physician's priorities).

Another powerful example of communicating care is through care of the environment. Every nurse knows that one cardinal way we communicate such tenets as comfort, respect, cleanliness/infection control, wellness/well-being, and safety to patients and their families is through appropriate care of the environment. Dirty linen, clutter, wrinkled or untidy bedding, trash, filth, or any kind or poor design of equipment and layout communicate "poor care given here," or "we don't care about you," or "we are so hassled and poorly organized, we don't have time to worry about such details," or "we don't respect ourselves or our work." This is a fundamental principle of communicating care that many contemporary nurses seem to overlook. What communication do you impart to clients in your work setting based on your care of the environment? The next time you walk into a client room or space, and the next time you walk onto the floor where you work, ask yourself, "What is communicated?" When you walk into your boss's office, into a meeting, or into anyone's office, take a moment to ask yourself, "What does this space say about these people?"

Nonverbal communication also comes in the form of personal appearance, gestures, and vibes. Remember the adage, "Who you are speaks so loudly that I can't hear what you are trying to say." Understanding cultural differences is also vital; a sleeveless blouse in Saudi Arabia is highly offensive, but a bikini in California is culturally appropriate. We communicate a potent message through our personal appearance: dress, neatness, hair style, make-up and nail care, jewelry, and shoes. Impressions—our first opportunities for communication—are made within the first 7 seconds; thereafter, our words either support or negate that impression, but impressions often get in the way of being heard. Wrinkled uniforms, messy or unkempt hair, worn, dirty shoes, and blatant make-up and nails or jewelry convey specific messages; personal expression is valued in our culture, but if that individualism communicates "I don't care about infection control" (dirty shoes), "I don't care about looking professional as you lie there looking to me for security and safety" (wrinkled, unkempt appearance), or "I don't care about your sensibilities" (bold make-up, nails, or jewelry), we communicate a potent message of disrespect for those we serve.

We can communicate many things by how we dress. Some managers dress in power suits and wear conservative standard make-up and jewelry; they conform to a style that is meant to be harsh, to emanate control—some feel the need to compete in a "man's world"—and to express power. Others may "dress down" to seem more open, casual, or friendly. Culture is expressed through attire and dress codes. What does your style of dress communicate? What do you want to communicate? What do you think nursing's contemporary identity communicates as a whole?

The next considerations of nonverbal communication are gestures and positioning. A position at the head of the table or a hand coming down firmly on the table offers a universally authoritative, even autocratic, message. Speaking with hands on hips or arms crossed while turning away from a client clearly communicates a combination of anger, impatience, lack of interest, and disrespect. Some communication is universally understood, whereas some communicators are culturally different. Holding hands during a conversation may convey respect and "I am connected to what you say" in some Middle Eastern cultures, whereas holding hands throughout a conversation in our Western culture may convey something very different. Although first impressions set the stage for our interactions, gestures and tone speak the loudest of all. As they say, it is all in the delivery.

We also communicate nonverbally through our mannerisms or actions. A gentle touch, warmed saline, and a warmed blanket provided during an abdominal dressing change imparts caring and respect for the patient. The use of time is a strong communicator. The way a task is completed imparts care, or the lack thereof. Hurriedly completing a procedure, rough actions, and inattention to details communicate "you are not worthy." Everything a nurse does with a patient—a client—either adds value or diminishes the value of that person and the value of care.

Positioning is another powerful communicator. Sit when you speak with a child; stand when an elder enters the room. As a speaker, guard yourself; hold yourself separate from the audience by standing behind the podium or walk around the stage. Sit at the head of the table or at the end of the table. Positioning is both one of our most powerful and potentially disempowering forms of communication. In today's healthcare arena, where is nursing positioned?

> *"Kindness in words creates confidence, kindness in thinking creates profoundness, kindness in giving creates love."*
> —Lao-Tzu

Think about how you respond to different styles. Does nursing need more power suits, different uniforms, greater standardization, or something else? What nonverbal communication must nursing develop and master? What environmental changes must the nursing profession address to produce effective managers and leaders? Is there a cookie cutter persona and environmental template, or does nursing need to communicate a whole new image? What is nursing's current brand? How do we look to the world?

Nonverbal communicators establish boundaries, construct barriers ("Do Not Enter"), and delineate rules (for the environment, rules such as "Employees Only" or personal style that bespeaks "stay away" or "I don't care"). The environmental design, care of the environment, and body language (attire, gestures, tone, mannerisms and actions, time, and positioning) are all compelling and potentially coercive communicators. What are you screaming loudly to the world without saying a word? As we look toward strategically aligning and planning nursing's future, we must be acutely aware of what we are currently communicating nonverbally and the many ways that we convey the meaning of care. We currently communicate a very poor brand; our current logo is "crisis."

VERBAL COMMUNICATION

Literacy—the ability to read and write—is necessary for effective verbal communication in our culture. Today, the constructs of communication literacy come in many forms—reading literacy, computer literacy, and technological literacy are just a few. The American Nurses Association's (ANA's) publication *Nursing: Scope and Standards of Practice* (2003) describes six communication competencies (literacy) for nurses: collaboration, collegiality, consultation, evaluation, leadership, and research. These literacy competencies are measured by the nurse's ability to communicate "with patient, family and healthcare providers regarding patient care and the nurse's role in the provision of that care" (collaboration); ability to share knowledge at care conferences/presentations and offering feedback (collegiality); ability to communicate "consultation recommendations that facilitate change" (consultation); ability to "disseminate the results to the patients and other involved" (evaluation); ability to promote communication of information and advancement of the profession through writing, publishing, and presentations" (leadership); and ability to "formally disseminate research findings" (research) (ANA, 2003). Each of these venues for communication is imperative to effectively aligning strategies in care.

Verbal communication is spoken, signed, or written, and is disseminated through the cacophony of available media forms (Internet, TV, DVDs, CDs, iPods, music, plays, journalism, research reports, education, satellites, radios, etc.). Culturally, we have a plethora of communication modalities that we are able to access; we may be proficient in some and lack expertise in others. Age, gender, and ethnicity all affect preferred methods of verbal communication (the so-called Y generation, for example, may be more comfortable and skilled with Internet technology, whereas the Baby Boomer generation may struggle to use computers).

Regardless of the modality, skill and understanding of verbal communicators are prerequisites to resetting the brand of nursing. How we say it is powerful (nonverbal), and what we say is pivotal. While the venue for the message

> *"The more elaborate our means of communication,*
> *the less we communicate."*
> —Diogenes Laërtius

depends on the audience, appropriate use of the media is critical; the media makes nurse's message possible. If nursing wants to reach teens, use the Internet; if nursing wants to reach seniors, use magazines and TV; if nursing wants to reach busy parents, use PDAs and iPods: How the message is delivered matters to those receiving the message. Pivotal, powerful, and possible communication are the tasks of the SP communicator.

What tone and body language are to spoken communication, punctuation, word choice, and brevity are to written communication. Exclamation points, vulgar language, and abruptness send a message of anger or disrespect; smiley faces, childish language, or excessive banter can send the same message in a different form. Emoticons, ☺ for example, are commonly used in e-mail messages and can be created using a combination of keystrokes.

Nurses' notes, electronic medical records, flow charts, and care plans are common communication tools for nurses, but are nurses proficient in professional communication? College nursing faculty must create portfolios that are submitted yearly for faculty review. Some employers require updated vitas and/or education records, but professional portfolios are not a standard expectation in nursing. Maintaining a professional portfolio is an essential communication tool for all nurses to strategically plan their career and to strategically align their career with their current position or the position they plan to achieve.

METACOMMUNICATION

Metacommunication is the message within the message. Sending messages—whether nonverbal or verbal—that are as clear as possible will facilitate the best possible results. Metacommunications come from behaviors such as manipulation, passive-aggressiveness, competition, hurt feelings, victimization, and a glut of dysfunctional drivers. People are feeling beings; we are motivated by our feelings, but that does not mean that we must be controlled by them. At the metacommunication level, there is the potential to create suppositions and innuendo. Feelings can become involved and the purpose of the communication can potentially be lost.

> *"The most important thing in communication is to hear what isn't being said."*
> —Peter Drucker, 1909–2005

You've heard the expression, "the straw that broke the camel's back." Communication is the tool set that we use to interact with life; communication is the process wherein many a straw has broken many a camel's back. Messages within messages are difficult to interpret; indeed, they have an array of possible interpretations, and they can be exhausting to try to figure out. Coffee break banter is filled with such interpretation puzzles.

Metacommunication can fuel angst, confusion, and hurt feelings. It can serve as a cultural subtlety necessary for communication. Metacommunication is ever present; it comes through the many forms of nonverbal and verbal messages. Unless it is a cultural imperative (such as saving face in the Indonesian culture), do your best to eliminate it from your communications, and do your best to seek clarification (again, as is culturally appropriate). Say what you mean and mean what you say, and if you don't get it right the first time, clarify; if you don't understand, ask for clarification.

Plans will never get off the ground if the team is mired in trying to figure out what the communicator is saying. Whether the communication is interpersonal, intrapersonal, or public, effectiveness is determined by the skill and knowledge of the communicator. There are four components of communication (see Table 10-1). These four tasks can get muddled or off track, or cause harm when nonverbal or verbal communication goes awry with metacommunication. The message and the feedback need to be clear, and the sender and receiver must be skilled in modalities of verbal and nonverbal cues for SP to be successfully communicated.

Communication is never linear (with just one path between sending and receiving). There are nine pathways to communicate within organizations (Table 10-2). The strategic planning communicator must be skilled in both the formal communication processes of his or her organization and be familiar with, and able to communicate through, the organization's informal (sometimes referred to as the grapevine) communication processes. This is often the most powerful stream of communication and is where messages are often mixed and inaptly interpreted.

Communication is a process that involves all available human senses. Effective communication is not simple, but it is essential in daily operation, especially during times of change. With the many modes, caveats, and pathways, communication is easily distorted; the role of the communicator in the strategic planning process cannot be underestimated. Architects and

Table 10-1   Components of Communication

1. Message
2. Sender
3. Receiver
4. Feedback

Table 10-2   Organizational Communication Pathways

1. Downward (top-down management)
2. Chain (leader is responsible for communication to others)
3. Y communication (leader to subordinates)
4. Wheel (leader at center of communication—communicates in several directions)
5. Circle (leader to others—report back to leader)
6. Upward (subordinates communicate up to leader)
7. Lateral (peer communication)
8. Diagonal (across departments or across agencies)
9. Grapevine (informal—multidirectional)

change agents require a vehicle to implementation; that vehicle is communication. Clear, energizing, and audience-appropriate communication facilitates transformational change designed by the architect and managed by the change agent.

SAY WHAT, SAY HOW? COMMUNICATION BASICS AND BARRIERS IN HEALTH CARE

Think before you speak. Know and understand your organization's formal and informal communication pathways. Become aware of your personal communication style and nonverbal communicators. Eliminate metacommunication. Employ audience-appropriate communicators and messages. Recognize and respect others' nonverbal styles. Respect cultural beliefs and practices. The cardinal rule to effective communication is best defined by Stephen Covey: Seek first to understand, and then to be understood (Covey, 1989).

There are many barriers to communication in today's healthcare environment. A recent *New York Times* article described dysfunctional interprofessional relationships. These communication patterns were cited as a contributing factor to poor retention rates in nursing and to creating chasms in quality care: "More often they [nurses] are belittled, insulted, even yelled at—often in front of patients and other staff members [by doctors]" (Tarkan, 2008). The article "Arrogant, Abusive and Disruptive—and a Doctor" discusses surveys of hospital staff members "who blame badly behaved doctors for low morale, stress and high turnover" (Tarkan, 2008); this is clearly unacceptable and ineffective. No one can effectively communicate when the sender or the receiver is behaving irrationally. The only logical response is to request that the person conduct himself or herself in a professional manner. Do not melt, do not cry, and do not fall into victim thinking. It never feels good to be yelled at, especially in public, but nursing must accept the fact that we have not only tolerated such horrid behavior, we have allowed it. Abusive behavior cannot exist if there is no one to abuse.

The majority of healthcare administrations are top-down, autocratic hierarchies dominated by men. The medical profession is male dominated. Although there is a distinct difference in some of the ways that men and women communicate, principles of professional communication can be learned by anyone. Nurses are competent interpersonal communicators; the competency that will facilitate empowered change in a business culture is the mastery of public communication. Technical writing, public speaking, and succinct verbal and nonverbal communication are some tools that will enable nurses to better participate in traditional business models.

DE BONO'S SIX WAYS TO SEE PERSPECTIVES AND STYLE

The role of the communicator is essential in supporting the architect and the change agent, but there is more to the communicator's job than just adhering to principles of sound professional communication; the communicator must also be cognizant of, and learn to align, what has been characterized as the six thinking hats (de Bono, 1999). People are not linear any more than communication is linear; people think about many things concurrently, and they can problem-solve in many dimensions simultaneously. Nurses do it all the time—noting and assessing wound odor, color, amount, and consistency of drainage while irrigating the wound and changing the dressing, then noting skin temperature, moisture, and color while questioning the client about pain, sensations, and comfort—all simultaneously. Several different cognitive, affective, and psychomotor abilities (or intelligences) come into play throughout a nurse's day.

In 1985, Harvard professor Edward de Bono identified a new way to think about how to think. The "Gang of Three," the Greek thinkers who influenced our Western thinking, comprise Socrates, Plato, and Aristotle. Their take on thinking was to point out what is wrong. This is one of the prevailing management paradigms today: Criticism leads to improvement, and pointing out what is wrong leads to fixing the problem. How does that work for you? How do you think that works for processes, systems, and projects? In addition to pointing out what is wrong, Socrates developed the notion that arguing about the problem led to discovering a solution. Does band-standing medication errors and then arguing about their causes fix them? The rate of prescribing medication errors did not change significantly between 1990 and 2002, remaining steady at 0.6 to 53 per 1000 (IOM, 2007). Tracking and arguing numbers does not address the human dynamic; human complexity problems require the multidimensional thinking inherent in parallel thought.

This is the basis of the scientific method, but it applies poorly to solving people problems. "Argument thinking," or traditional thinking, is one valid approach to understanding phenomena, but it does not allow for a holistic view of human dynamics and problem-solving. Argument thinking seeks to compartmentalize a phenomenon, to prove what is and what has been; in the end, someone must be right, and someone must be wrong.

Medical diagnoses obviously fit well with this model of thinking as it is based on the scientific method. For example, a nurse sees a patient with a headache. She conducts an assessment to determine etiology. Related to high blood pressure—why, why not? Related to injury—why, why not? Or related to medication, heat, dehydration, blood sugar, etc.—why, why not? From this process, the nurse will drill down to the "related to" and derive the appropriate nursing diagnosis. Argument thinking is useful in this scenario, but we have used this model of thinking for every process as a way to "judge our way forward" (de Bono, 1999, p. 3).

de Bono (1999) asserted that we must "design our way forward" (p. 3). de Bono's research demonstrated that a different type of thinking leads to supportive communication across the management and leadership process. He coined the term *parallel thinking* to describe this approach. Parallel thinking draws its influence from "what can be . . . constructive thinking, creative thinking" (p. 2). This "design forward" is a perfect match for strategic planning.

The overall principle of parallel thinking is that there are no opposites or confrontational points of view because all stakeholders look in the same direction. This does not suggest that everyone involved will think the same thoughts, but they will all be looking forward to address the phenomena instead of trying to compete or win.

de Bono[1] used the analogy of colored hats to describe how varying outlooks can be combined and strengthened. These hats do not define or categorize how a person thinks; remember, people are not linear. The six hats represent directions of thinking, to set out to think in a specific direction. People do have differing intelligences, strengths, and talents, but they are also capable of applying the necessary specific intelligences singularly. See Table 10-3 for de Bono's colored hats analogy.

---

[1]To learn more about parallel thinking please see Edward de Bono, *Six Thinking Hats* (1999).

Table 10-3   de Bono's Colored Hats

* White: neutral and objective—concerned with facts and figures
* Red: anger and emotions—the emotional view
* Black: somber, careful, and cautious—the weakness of the idea view
* Yellow: sunny and positive—the optimistic view
* Green: like grass, abundant—the creative view
* Blue: color of the sky, the big picture—the overview

Thinking about the wound example, the nurse used many hats. The assessment process began with objective data (amount, odor, color, temp, etc.): white hat. The emotions may have been engaged if the nurse experienced empathy for the patient's trials and discomfort: red hat. Caution may have been necessary to weigh differing irrigation or dressing approaches: black hat. Anticipating a healed wound, assuring the patient of progress, and imparting a positive attitude to support the patient: yellow hat. Even the most routine dressing changes can have caveats; sterile gauze that has knotted in the bottle, forceps that lock, a sterile package that won't open correctly—all require creative problem-solving: green hat. And finally, a panoramic patient assessment is always done before leaving the room: blue hat.

Parallel thinking goes beyond categories of thought or problem-solving. Parallel thinking is a practical and positive approach to exploring new ideas and making decisions; parallel thinking is strategic thinking. Traditional argument thinking leads to confusion and can be weighted by dominance; those with power usually win arguments or discussions. And traditional thinking can be hierarchical and elitist.

The profession of nursing has long been guided by the folly of employing only traditional thinking to nurses' organizational challenges and chasms. Advanced practice (AP) nurses and nurse practitioners (NPs) view nursing problems through their specific lenses; some of the worst treatment (finding fault, accusing of error, judging forward) of staff nurses comes from APs and NPs. Nurse administrators often operate from a similar paradigm; administration is right, and errors are committed by staff nurses who are wrong. Each level and discipline of nursing has been looking through individual lenses. de Bono's parallel thinking would have nursing join all levels and disciplines together to work together to design forward. All of nursing wears the same hat to solve a problem. The hats change as the problem need changes (see Table 10-4).

Table 10-4   Changing Hats

1. Starting with yellow, nurses design an ideal vision of care.
2. Move to all wearing a white hat to conduct a strategic review.
3. Hurt, anger, or other emotions may need to be aired and explored—on goes the red hat for every nurse.
4. Then move to the strategic thinking and creative solutions. Everybody grab a green hat and design strategies to heal care and remove the giant scarlet C.
5. Time to review and consider the strengths and weaknesses of the plan—on with the black hat.
6. Now it is time to take a broader view. Look at the plan from every angle—a 360° view. Every nurse wears a blue hat.

THE LEADER WITHIN: HAVE YOU MET? PRINCIPLES VERSUS TECHNIQUE

Managers are everywhere, but leaders are harder to come by. As Dr. Steven Covey and Peter Drucker[2] succinctly submit, you manage things and you lead people We've discussed management versus leadership many times throughout this text because the concepts are critical to whether nursing will be able to make the quantum change that is necessary to solve the shortage and the errors, chasms, and disparities in care. Designing a way forward can only be accomplished by self-leadership and self-management. Every day, nurses choose—disgruntled or content, weak or empowered, victim or change agent, positive or negative, blamer or accepting of responsibility. "Significant, sustainable quality must ultimately be generated inside-out" (Covey, 1995, ¶#1). Each nurse has the ability to create significant, sustainable quality in care. We recognize the need for change. Each nurse must decide if he or she wants to stay with the status quo or design forward. The only sustainable path to quality improvement in nursing—in care—is paved by principles.

> *"There are three constants in life . . . change, choice and principles."*
> —Dr. Stephen R. Covey, 1932–Present

[2]Peter Drucker was a business leader and is the author of many books on management and business; he is known as the inventor of modern management.

There is a variety of techniques that might describe care—competencies, evidence-based practice, benchmarks—all based on various techniques (argument thinking). The principles that circumscribe nursing are the principles that define care: Principles such as dignity, respect, compassion, altruism, charity, tolerance, inquiry, compassion, ethics, morality, and excellence then drive the techniques that are identified as nursing. When the correct principles are engrained in the profession of care—professionally understood and adopted—the techniques (skills, practices, and beliefs) are naturally founded in quality (parallel thinking). Principles based on clear values are easily muddled in today's fast-paced healthcare arena. Leadership flows from principles; management flows from techniques. Have you been technique driven or principle driven?

Take a moment to stop and ask yourself what the guiding principles are for you as a nurse and get reacquainted with the leader within. You knew her when you started your nursing career; it is time to reclaim the core of nursing and the principles of care as we all design new strategies to heal the profession (parallel thinking). We will not continue to belabor the point that management manages things and leaders lead people, but the distinction is paramount as you think about your individual career and the profession as a whole. It is of interest that most of the strategies developed by the Institute of Medicine, the Department of Health and Human Services, and related agencies to address quality of care are techniques. Nursing is in as great a crisis as it was 10 years ago; techniques have not been the answer.

> Management comes after leadership; leadership drives strategic planning; management helps keep it on task.

"True leadership . . . has never been a matter of formal authority. Leaders are effective when the people around them acknowledge them as leaders. A title does not make a leader; a real leader is set apart by his or her attributes, attitudes, and behaviors" (Harvard Business School Press, 2004, p. 200). Historically, the practice of nursing has been based on management techniques. Leadership, as an inside job, will design the way forward.

A NOTE ON "STRATEGIC THINKING"

In Chapter 2, we talked about the fuzzy thinking that has led to our current realities in care. Suzanne Gordon, a journalist, was able to diagnose nursing's ills without ever having stepped in a nursing classroom: denursification. "As a man [or woman] thinketh in his heart, so he [she] is" (Proverbs 23:10). What does our state of nursing tell you about nursing's heart? If this centuries-old proverb is true, then there is a mighty lack of the right kind of thinking in nursing. Nursing has been looking in so many directions from an argument technique vantage that making some premise, level, or practice right and one wrong has become the cultural norm—this is inadequate thinking.

We want to offer you a note here about strategic thinking. As you have studied this text, we hope that you have gained an appreciation for an expanded worldview of nursing and business and to question the paradigms that encapsulate nursing. Imagine—strategically think about—no power struggles, no blame, no elitism, just an empowered nursing workforce engaged in solving the crisis together. This would be strategic thinking in nursing at its best—every nurse looking in the same direction and designing a way forward (de Bono, 1999).

WHAT'S WITH THIS MEETING ANYWAY? MEETING ETIQUETTE

Strategic planning requires meetings. Depending on the scope of the plan, perhaps several meetings each week may be necessary. Managers from one major New York investment corporation meet 8–10 hours every day. Possessing meeting etiquette and understanding the various types of meetings are skills that no one ever teaches; people are automatically expected to know how to function within meetings. If you have time to read about meetings, there are books galore on meeting styles and purpose, how to conduct a meeting, who should attend, and how to form teams and create buy-in. There are only two principles of meetings that are universal: Do not meet unless it is necessary to have a group decision or process, and do not meet without a set agenda that all participants have had the opportunity to review, consider, and offer input on— what's termed objective driven.

Meetings can be tremendous time wasters that create confusion, inflate egos, separate "workers" from "the meeting organizers," increase workloads, and take away from productivity. As social beings, most people like meetings, their status, and/or the opportunity to express ideas or opinions, or people may use meetings as a default setting, just what we do. Some meetings flow from crisis, some from routine (Monday morning meetings), some from collaboration, and some from reward or punishment; some seem to have no purpose whatsoever. Strategic planning will require meetings: meetings to set vision, define values, and create mission; meetings to assess strengths and weaknesses, threats and opportunities; meetings to manage resources; meetings to facilitate implementation; meetings to evaluate progress; and meetings to create sustainability. Nurses need to function optimally as meeting members, facilitators, or leaders.

All meetings will have a specific purpose and an agenda for which everyone has had ample time to review and offer comments. Table 10-5 lists basic rules for conducting meetings.

Meetings should be objective driven, pleasant, and productive. You want participants to be fully engaged, offer their best ideas, come prepared, and be

---

Table 10-5   Basic Meeting Rules

- Address the highest priority first.
- Limit the topics based on available time.
- Avoid getting sidetracked; stick to the items on the agenda.
- Be prepared with necessary data or materials.
- Have enough handouts for all attendees.
- Assign a facilitator or chair.
- Assign a timekeeper to keep the meeting within the scheduled time frame.
- Assign a scribe or minutes person.
- Consider implementing parliamentary procedure: Parliamentary procedure exists to "facilitate the transaction of business and to promote cooperation and harmony" (Cagle, 2009). All attendees have equal privileges, rights, and obligations. The majority decides; minorities have rights to be protected; a quorum (minimum number) has to be present; there will be full and unencumbered discussion of all matters or motions; only one question or topic is considered at a time; everyone must know and understand points before voting; no member speaks until acknowledged by the chair or facilitator; everyone has an opportunity to speak; the speaker has the floor; chair or facilitator remains impartial.
- Schedule meeting time accordingly, avoiding hours of heavy workload, late afternoons, holidays, times near deadlines, or when the flu is going through the hospital.
- Snacks, coffee, tea, and water are only necessary for meetings that extend beyond 2 hours.
- Limit breaks to 10 minutes approximately every hour.
- Start and end on time.
- Always leave 5–10 minutes to summarize decisions, action steps, and responsibilities.
- Set up and test IT equipment *before* the meeting.
- Create a comfortable meeting environment (chairs, tables, temperature control).
- Provide meeting minutes within the same workweek to all participants.
- Schedule the next meeting before adjourning.
- Ask for future agenda items; include this information in the minutes, along with the next meeting date, time, and location.

willing (and wanting) to participate again. The purpose of a meeting is group communication. Gathering people to listen to a lecture does not provide a sound reason to meet; lecture-type communication is better delivered via memos, Web links, or e-mails—or, better yet, not delivered at all (adults are better served using parallel thinking techniques during meetings).

Meetings can take a few minutes to several hours or days depending on the scope and intent of the process. The strategic planning process requires effective communication across all departments and with all stakeholders. Be clear about the meeting's intent, and the appropriate process and setting will follow. A meeting that is meant to redesign the nursing unit's vision and mission statement would not fit a parliamentary process. A meeting that discusses budgets probably shouldn't be held in a casino. A meeting whose purpose is to engage strategic thinking needs time and tools that might best be facilitated in a retreat venue. Begin with the purpose in mind, and the flow and structure will follow; form follows function.

REMEMBER YOUR GOAL, EXCELLENCE IN CARE: ALL THE OTHER STUFF IS JUST STUFF

Communication is a human experience. No matter how skilled or how proficient, people can be messy communicators, communication breaks down, and communication strategies fail. But then dealing with people, wherever and whenever, can be messy and frustrating. We try to hide or eliminate metacommunication, but it shows up anyway. Expressed emotions from one source seem to allow other unrelated emotions to tumble out too. Because change is often threatening, remember that people are security-seeking organisms. Strategic planning asks people to step out of their comfort zones and design and implement a new culture. And when a person's security is threatened, anger is often the first emotion that pops up. Threatened individuals can create tremendous barriers to change. And the more power that person has, the greater the impact.

People have power through several paths. The screaming doctor has power because he or she claims it, and no one stops or challenges the behavior; power can be claimed through intimidation and abuse. A second pathway to power is earned by virtue of attributes, skill, and intelligence. Power can also be purchased; money can buy power. Power comes from strengthening others; benefiting others benefits the one. Power may come from virtues or idealized characteristics. People with talents, such as athletic ability, have power. Certain personalities can be domineering and claim power in meetings. One form of power that can undermine a process is the popularity power. Strong personalities, quick wit, and sharp tongues can dominate processes. Claiming power culturally implies aggression and dominance, but it need not. Power is not evil, nor should it harm anyone or anything. How would you like to see nursing claim its power? How can you claim your power?

Knowing whom you are working with—and where the power grids reside— is key to effective strategic planning processes. Getting people to design forward, communicate efficiently and effectively, and participate in meetings that run like the well-greased gears of a magnificent machine is not a simple task.

Nursing has many communication skills in its toolbox, but the role of communicator in strategic planning requires that nursing acquire communication skills and techniques used in business. Instead of thinking from a blame or argument stance, nursing will be well served to engage in parallel thinking. The goal of any and all nursing types and settings is excellence in care. When we understand the array and cacophony that is communication, we are better equipped to be patient, understanding, and able to solve interpersonal and public communication challenges. There is a lot to human interactions. The strategic planning communicator navigates the territory to reach the goal: an empowered nursing workforce devoid of the scarlet C.

See Appendix 10 to calculate your communication quotient.

REVIEW QUESTIONS

1. Unkempt appearance is an example of what type of communication?
2. List five examples of nonverbal communication expressed through the care of the environment.
3. List the ANA's six communication competencies for nurses.
4. What form of communication is writing?
5. What are the four components of communication?
6. List four examples of metacommunication.
7. Compare parallel communication and traditional communication.

REFERENCES

American Nurses Association (ANA). (2003). *Nursing: Scope and standard of practice.* Silver Spring, MD: NursesBooks.org.

Cagle, J. A. (2009). *Parliamentary procedure: Toward the good order of the university.* Retrieved January 13, 2009, from http://www.csufresno.edu/comm/cagle-p3.htm

Covey, S. R. (1989). *The 7 habits of highly effective people.* New York: Fireside Books.

Covey, S. R. (1995). *Principle-centered leadership: Sharpen the saw.* Retrieved January 12, 2009, from http://www.qualitydigest.com/nov95/html/prin-cnt.html

de Bono, E. (1999). *Six thinking hats*. New York: Little, Brown & Co.

Harvard Business School Press. (2004). *Harvard business essentials: Manager's toolkit: The 13 skills managers need to succeed*. Boston: Author.

Institute of Medicine (IOM), Committee on Identifying and Preventing Medication Errors, Board on Health Care Services. (2007). *Preventing medication errors: Quality chasm series*. Washington, DC: National Academies Press.

Kaplan, R., & Norton, D. (1996). *The Balanced Scorecard: Translating strategy into action*. Boston: Harvard Business School Press.

Tarkan, L. (2008, December 2). Arrogant, abusive and disruptive—and a doctor. *The New York Times*. Retrieved December 2, 2008, from http://www.nytimes.com/2008/12/02/health/02rage.html

Calculate Your Communication Quotient

The first aspect of communication quotients is professional appearance (recall that 7 seconds equals the first impression). We would like you to stand in front of a full-length mirror and assess what your general appearance, including hygiene, communicates:

1 = respectful, clean   2 = some people think I look OK   3 = I don't care

Your quotient: _____

Second, talk in front of the mirror and watch how you use your hands, your facial gestures, and the stance you use:

1 = nonthreatening, gentle   2 = a little assertive   3 = aggressive

Your quotient: _____

Next, ask someone who knows you well what mannerisms or quirks you have:

1 = calm, attentive   2 = little movements, little fidgets   3 = like talking to a jumping bean

Your quotient: _____

How many um, ya know, like, awesome, geez, and other slang or distracting words or phrases do you use?

1 = rarely   2 = sometimes   3 = like, totally, dude

Your quotient: _____

Your written communication is:

1 = articulate/well written   2 = average, a little confusing   3 = spelling/grammar nightmare

Your quotient: ____

When problem-solving, do you prefer to hash it out and argue the points, and feel the need to establish a "right" and a "wrong" solution?

1 = prefer creative solutions   2 = depends on the problem   3 = absolutely

Your quotient: _____

In a meeting, you:

1 = are prepared/participate   2 = sometimes fall asleep   3 = go for the donuts

Your quotient: _____

Add up your quotients: 7–10 is a higher communication quotient ability than 11–21. If you have a 21, we kindly suggest that you reevaluate your communication style—at least in the business setting. Don't stop being yourself, and do not compromise your values, but effective communication will help all of us to design our way forward through the strategic planning process.

Eight Pitfalls of Strategic Planning

A little history lesson from past planning exercises: Do you see yourself, your sphere of influence, or any of the cardinal team members in any of the "eight cautionary tales"? Honestly, what is the potential buy-in? Is it a little brick wall, or are we talking the Great Wall of China? The size and scope of the undertaking may be too big. Who will the architect be? Who will the communicator be? Who will the change agent be? (*Choose wisely, grasshopper . . .*) This chapter takes a clear look at the pitfalls of the strategic planning process: what is working and what isn't; what has been derailing nursing's power; why derailments exist; and how and when to reassess, redesign, or abandon the process.

COMPLEXITY OVERLOAD AND DECISION-MAKING SHORTCUTS

"We're going to eliminate errors and waste, and we are going to do it in three easy steps over the next 4 days using staff whom we don't have to pay benefits, and equipment that can be fixed with duct tape." This may seem ridiculous, but unfortunately strategic plans exist that ask people and systems to take on more work without realistic and necessary support. "We need you to be a team player" is one of the more common motivating techniques when infrastructure is insufficient to support desired results. The design and implementation of a strategic plan requires that resources be realistically assessed and continually monitored throughout change management processes.

"Silo-ing" (Gentile, 2008) refers to artificial and often counterproductive separation of management and staff. Silo-ing creates a division between the many stakeholders of care: staff in one silo, managers/administration in a separate silo, patients or clients in yet another. In the design stages of the strategic planning (SP) process, perpetuation of "management by silos" leads to unrealistic strategic thinking and plans, complexity overload, and decision-making shortcuts. Even the simplest designs become complex when they reach the implementation stage if resources are not adequately evaluated and respected.

A poignant example of this in nursing was the decision to improve nursing's image and autonomy by creating more nurse managers. A few managers developed the idea for many within a silo. The results: alienation and competition across levels of nursing were created, bedside care was devalued, and patient outcomes were negatively affected. The need for nurse managers is a sound and necessary premise. The strategy was not the problem; the problem was created because the strategy was created in a silo, the complexity of the change was not thoroughly investigated (using situational analysis), the design was too Byzantine, and the shortcuts led to the "we need you to be a team player" approach to implementation management. Today, nurse managers walk a tenuous tightrope between the interests of nurses (care) and the interests of business (profit) as BSN preparation has evolved to emphasize management instead of bedside care—a dysfunctional position generated by inadequate strategic thinking and planning. Ohmae (1988) sees this SP shortfall through the analogy of approaching strategic planning with the "tip of the iceberg" avenue, addressing only what is visible.

It was obvious that nursing needed to work more closely with administration, but as Suzanne Gordon (2005) so aptly summarized in *Nursing Against the Odds*, "In spite of hospital rhetoric evincing a newfound concern for the value of nurses, nurses have had to wage bruising strikes to get modest increases in wages, safe nurse-to-patient ratios, an end to mandatory overtime, the implementation of predictable schedules, and a modicum of voice in institutional policies that govern their work" (p. 5). Adding more nurse managers became a Band Aid for a hemorrhage. Complexity overload and solution shortcuts are the result of insufficient attention to the strategic review: Pitfall #1.

HAIL, HAIL, THE GANG IS *NOT* ALL HERE

Buy-in is an elusive concept. People may declare cooperation and interest pub-
lically but undermine change efforts covertly. As described in the first section,
silo-ing creates this conundrum: Ohmae (1988) described this pitfall to SP as
"failing to collaborate with staff" and "losing sight of the member" (in this case,
nurses). "Because strategy creation is a complex, drawn-out affair, it is dis-
tressingly easy to lose sight of what matters most: the member" (Liff, 2008).
The primary principle to buy-in is to establish communication pathways and
feedback loops that build buy-in.

Kotter (1996) set eight stages to creating buy-in and making sure that the
"gang is all here":

1. Establish a sense of urgency—a compelling reason to address change
   (strategic planning).
2. Create a guiding coalition (SP team).
3. Develop a vision and a strategy that is feasible.
4. Articulately and succinctly communicate the vision to all stakeholders
   (better yet, have all stakeholders participate in the visioning process).
5. Empower employees (Kotter described four traditional barriers to empowerment: formal structures, bosses' interference/discouragement, clogged
   personnel and information systems, and lack of necessary skills).
6. Generate short-term wins (discussed later in this chapter).
7. Consolidate gains and produce more change (major change takes a long
   time; celebrate short-term wins, but do not lose sight of the bigger
   vision; a focus on minutiae can lead to a loss of urgency).
8. Anchor new strategies in the culture (acknowledging change as an end
   point does not equate with sustainable change; significant change must
   be sustainable).

A fundamental principle of working with adults is that in order to effectively engage them in any process, they must understand the meaning as it is
relevant to them. Top-down autocratic dogma works with exclusively industry processes to some extent, but contemporary management and leadership
research consistently demonstrates that today's knowledge worker can,
wants to, and must participate in decision-making processes. A simple review
of nursing conferences and workshops demonstrates the breach of this principle. "Nurse leaders decide" is a common subtitle as small groups of self-
appointed nursing "leaders" have determined that they represent 15 million
nurses; not unlike the "good-old boys" clubs of medicine and administration,
nursing has created some of its own "good old nurses" clubs that are disconnected from care.

Buy-in is all about respect. Nurses are in one of the easiest professions to change, given the right motivators and rationale. As with no other profession, nursing is based on care; the ethics and morals that drive a person to want to practice care are always available as a tool to effect change. If leaders and mangers want to create buy-in from nurses, the solution is very simple: Demonstrate how the change will improve care and strengthen the role of the nurse. Time management, cost-effectiveness, and improved (lessened) patient turnaround times do not motivate nurses; empowered autonomous quality care does. Failing to achieve consensus is Pitfall #2.

FUZZY VISION IN A DARK ROOM

Strategic change processes are supposed to begin with a clear vision that is communicated effectively. We've asked you in earlier chapters to define your vision for nursing and to describe what you think the current vision for nursing is both nationally and worldwide. Combined, the authors have worked in nursing for 49 years, and we cannot tell you what our national "leaders" see for nursing's future. Recently the American Nurses Association (ANA) released the "BSN in 10" (Trossman, 2008). However that is not a vision but a technique. Pay for performance, Magnet Status, and many other strategies are advanced to address the scarlet C, but a clear design of the way forward has yet to be articulated in a unified voice that represents all nurses. There are vision statements for advanced practice (AP), nursing education, and levels of practice. The only unified vision for care comes from the International Council of Nurses (ICN) in Geneva, Switzerland:

> United within ICN, the nurses of all nations speak with one voice. We speak as advocates for all those we serve, and for all the unserved, insisting that prevention, care and cure be the right of every human being. We are in the vanguard of health care progress, shaping health policy around the world through our expertise, the strength of our numbers, the alignment of our efforts, and our collaboration with the public and with other health professionals.
>
> Our mission is to lead our societies toward better health. Working together within ICN, we harness the knowledge and enthusiasm of the entire nursing profession to promote healthy lifestyles, healthy workplaces, and healthy communities. We foster the health of our societies as well as individuals by supporting strategies of sustainable development that mitigate poverty, pollution, and other underlying causes of illness.
>
> Working together, we are at the forefront of incorporating advanced technology into health care without losing the human element. We are determined that science and technology remain the servant of compassionate and ethical caring that includes meeting spiritual and emotional needs.

Working together, and reaching out to involve nursing students, we are achieving higher levels of nursing education in every nation—education that is liberally and scientifically based, flexible and culturally sensitive, and founded on the core values of our profession. We ensure that nurses are educated for broad provider and policy roles that fully integrate and utilize nursing within multidisciplinary health teams. We equip nurses to be skilled points of entry for health care, able to care for clients and to guide them to other care givers as appropriate. We continually add new clusters of competencies to lead and reflect dynamic changes in health care, and we insure that health care systems recognize and reward those competencies. Together, we work for values, policies, standards and conditions that free nurses to practice to the full extent of their education and ability. Our work together is guided by a common philosophy of nursing: a commitment to caring in the fullest sense, being advocates for our patients, helping people to help themselves, and doing for people what they would do unaided if they had the necessary strength, will, or knowledge . . . Approved by the Board of Directors; ICN; November 1998. (ICN, 2009)

This is the closest thing to a vision statement that we could find for the ANA:

The American Nurses Association (ANA) is the only full-service professional organization representing the nation's 2.9 million registered nurses (RNs) through its 54 constituent member associations. The ANA advances the nursing profession by fostering high standards of nursing practice, promoting the rights of nurses in the workplace, projecting a positive and realistic view of nursing, and by lobbying the Congress and regulatory agencies on health care issues affecting nurses and the public. (ANA, 2009)

The National League for Nursing (NLN) has set four goals for nursing education that have embedded visions:

Leader in Nursing Education—Enhance the NLN's national and international impact as the recognized leader in nursing education.
Commitment to Members—Build a diverse, sustainable, member-led organization with the capacity to deliver our mission effectively, efficiently, and in accordance with our values.
Champion for Nurse Educators—Be the voice of nurse educators and champion their interests in political, academic, and professional arenas.
Advancement of the Science of Nursing Education—Promote evidence-based nursing education and the scholarship of teaching. (NLN, 2009)

The statements from these organizations are clear, but the ICN best articulates a vision for all of nursing regardless of level and discipline, and across borders. Take out your vision statement and see how your view aligns with these three. Schools of nursing, clinics, hospitals, nursing centers, and almost every setting where care is practiced have developed their own vision statement; are they in line with that of the ICN? Nursing must have a clear vision that all nurses can see in order to design a way forward, lest a common pitfall to SP be exacerbated—being mired in fuzzy thinking: Pitfall #3.

I CAN SEE JUST FINE; I FORGOT THAT YOU WEAR CORRECTIVE LENSES

Filters to perception come in many forms; culture, gender, literacy, experience, worldview, attitudes, education, and the environment are just a few factors that can alter or impair vision. Because of these filters, some people will need corrective lenses to create buy-in and facilitate change. Our beliefs interpret what we see—contrary to the notion that if we teach everyone the same thing in the same way, everyone will arrive at the same conclusion. Recall de Bono and the six hats, the cacophony of communication styles and methods, the three general types of learning (cognitive, psycho-motor, and affective), and the multiple intelligences of humanity developed by Howard Gardner in 1983.[1] People, their personalities, cultures, and backgrounds are unique. It isn't that they are incapable of engaging in strategic planning and change processes; they just may be coming to the table with fresh perspectives, or they may function more effectively if they are given the opportunity to learn and understand the processes and drivers. A common pitfall of SP is to assume that one message fits all: Pitfall #4.

ABSENCE OF PLANNING SHORT-TERM RESULTS OR NOT RECOGNIZING THEM: THERE IS MORE THAN ONE GOLDEN RING!

Motivation is a subject all its own, but suffice it to say people operate from different levels and needs for gratification. Although some are motivated by long-term gratification, the human mind is a solution-seeking organism and, as such, usually derives motivation from short-term wins. Change is a sometimes difficult process that can take weeks, months, or years. In the day-to-day press of responsibilities, vision and strategic plans can get lost in the shuffle; many a wonderful strategic plan has ended up on a dusty shelf.

Part of the solution to forward motion is a sound plan and a dedicated and skilled team. One simple tool to keep plans on track is to design short-term wins (progress measures) into the process. A hospital bulletin board offers a

---

[1]Linguistic intelligence ("word smart"); logical-mathematical intelligence ("number/reasoning smart"); spatial intelligence ("picture smart"); bodily-kinesthetic intelligence ("body smart"); musical intelligence ("music smart"); interpersonal intelligence ("people smart"); intrapersonal intelligence ("self smart"); and naturalist intelligence ("nature smart").

pizza party when 365 error-free days are reached. First, pizza is not a great adult motivator, and second, 365 days is too far out there. Choose appropriate motivators that are time sensitive and appropriate: Many a golden watch given at retirement is tossed in a drawer, a mockery of what it is meant to represent.

SP should be broken into realistic, manageable, and coherent components and be tied to appropriate motivators. Some motivation can come in the form of "atta girls," but words must match action. Nurses being told that they are doing a great job in decreasing medication errors while simultaneously being criticized for not working more hours will not see the golden ring and will most likely lose interest in the change process. Another common pitfall is the assumption that original buy-in will sustain the process. Absence of planning for short-term results and rewards can take the steam out of the original enthusiasm and momentum: Pitfall #5.

ROADBLOCKS—AND NO WAY AROUND (OR SO YOU THINK!)

Roadblocks and challenges are a part of life. As the saying goes, life happens. In Chapter 4, we discussed the need for a contingency plan. Emergency plans exist for most organizations: "What to do if . . ." The same principle of preparedness is necessary for an SP. In fact, much of the contingency plan can be adopted from the organization's emergency plan. However, some variables must be addressed as they arise. The financial crisis that began in 2008 revealed that many companies had less viable SPs or no SP; they were caught in a dramatic economic downturn with no way to respond. Some eventualities do spell disaster for an organization, even with the best contingency plan. Plans cannot address every eventuality, but roadblocks do not necessarily mean "stop here"; they usually imply "detour ahead."

> *"The one thing that he [we] can try is to find, and occasionally create, the right risk and to exploit uncertainty."*
> —Peter Drucker, 1909–2005

Roadblocks and delays can cause team members and participants to lose heart and become discouraged. The strategic liaison, or change agent, needs to keep on top of the shifting personalities of change. Monday, everyone is charged up, on task, and on schedule. Tuesday, a snowstorm hits; power is lost to half the city, and employees are struggling with frozen pipes, unsafe driving conditions, and finding batteries. By Thursday, the first round of flu bugs hits, and staffing is the primary concern. Three weeks later, things begin to stabilize, but the change process has to start back where it had been the last Monday—a few steps backward and a few more forward. An automated assembly line that is automated can work with predictable precision, but roadblocks come up when the necessary implementation resource is people. Built-in flexibility in contingency plans, emergency plans, and strategic plans helps to address "life"; as priorities shift, competent leadership and management are prepared to respond. The real issue with roadblocks is not the deterrent itself; it is the capability and capacity of management, leadership, and the strategic planning team to surmount roadblocks and make necessary adaptations. The real pitfall on the road through strategic planning involves how well leaders and managers navigate detours: Pitfall #6.

THIS ISN'T REALLY THE FINISH LINE—DON'T CELEBRATE TOO SOON

Pitfall #5 is failing to reward short-term wins, but it is also a dilemma to have a fuzzy finish line and fizzle out. These pitfalls are all tied together. Most tie into the clarity and compulsion of the vision statement and the strategic planning team's ability to keep everyone's eyes on the prize. Short-term wins and motivators are crucial to modifying human behavior. But if overemphasized, they can lead to cultural complacency. The change agent is very busy during these transitional periods in the planning progress.

Let's use the example of total quality improvement (TQI) on a medical surgical unit. TQI encapsulates every variable that measures patient outcomes. For this example, let's look at the "never events" established in the Centers for Medicare and Medicaid (CMS) Deficit Reduction Act (DRA) of 2005 (CMS, 2009a; 2009b). The potential exists to assess 12 different outcome measures as defined by the never events.

The staff and infection control personnel have identified a 30% incidence of urinary tract infections associated with indwelling urinary catheters. Management is motivated to eliminate these infections because CMS will no longer pay for costs associated with these types of infections, and the nursing staff are motivated because the patients' well-being and recovery rates are affected. Strategies to decrease this type of infection are driven by evidence-based practice (EBP) and include strategies such as fewer catheterization days, fewer indwelling catheters inserted, strict attention to sterile technique and aseptic technique, improved screening prior to insertion, and improved staff education and audits (Angelo, 2007).

The medical-surgical staff implement these strategies, and indwelling urinary catheter infection rates drop by 62%. Achieving this benchmark saves money, improves patient outcomes, and is a deeply gratifying motivator for the nursing staff. Such a rate reduction requires a sound strategic plan, time, energy, and expended resources, but it is only one piece of the TQI strategic plan to eliminate all CMS never events.

The change agent and the communicator must be skilled in delivering the golden rings, not declare success too soon, and keep all stakeholders energized to see the next piece of the TQI process that is outlined in the SP. After-all, SP is a tool to actualize quality. Quality is not an end mark; quality is a process that evolves with EBP and research. Strategic planning, like TQI, is not stationary; just as with the CMS example, there are more events to attend to. Don't declare, "We've crossed the finish line" too soon: Pitfall #7.

CHANGE THAT IS A SQUARE PEG IN A ROUND HOLE: CULTURE ALIGNMENT AND CORPORATE ALIGNMENT— WOW, CAN THEY EVER COLLIDE!

If you are a square peg trying to fit into a round hole, one of two things must happen: Your paradigm needs to shift to being round, or you need to quit trying to align what doesn't align. As difficult as it is, sometimes the best strategy is simply to walk away. The only compass that we can offer you for this Herculean undertaking is to honestly determine value alignment. Are your values in alignment with those of your organization? Is there a reasonable path (avoiding battlefields and casualties) that can affect value shifts? The answer is not to swallow your values and stick it out. Nor is it to stay, be miserable, and share your misery. You now have an idea how to navigate a change process professionally. If you do not have the desire, energy, or support to instigate the change that you wish to see, you also have two choices: grin and bear it, or find a cultural fit elsewhere.

You may have the most brilliant, ethical, and responsive strategic solutions for TQI, but some organizations are so clogged with atherosclerotic dysfunction plied by layers of hierarchy that you will need to be infinitely patient or outlive everybody else. One pitfall, fortunately not common, is a poor fit: Pitfall #8.

LET'S THINK ABOUT YOUR STRATEGIC PLANNING EXPERIENCE: SUCCESSES, FAILURES, STRENGTHS, AND WEAKNESSES—HAVE YOU FALLEN PREY TO STRATEGIC PLANNING'S PITFALLS?

Before we leave the subject of barriers to strategic planning, let's take another glance over our shoulder to past experiences with SP. Now that you have an expanded view of the strategic planning process, take a moment to evaluate your past experiences and why you considered them successful or not:

Experiences with SP:

When:_____ Where:_____

    Purpose:_____

    Participants:_____

    Leaders:_____

    Outcome:_____

    Your perceptions +/–:_____

    Why (pitfalls)?_____

    _____

Strengths:

    What were the plan's strengths?_____

    _____

Weaknesses:

    What were the plan's weaknesses?_____

    _____

    How could the pitfalls or weaknesses have been avoided?_____

    _____

    _____

A FEW WORDS ABOUT THE WORD *FAILURE*

Don't use it. It is as simple as that. The word *failure* can refer to an IV pump, but it has no home in the realm of human interaction, actions, assessments, or value judgments. As Thomas Edison said about discovering the light bulb, "I have not failed. I've just found 10,000 ways that won't work."

Strategic planning, change, or improvement initiatives will run into some of the aforementioned pitfalls; perhaps you have identified or experienced other pitfalls. "Failure is not an option" is not a statement about the action of failing; it is a statement of impossibility. People cannot fail; they can quit, they can become frustrated, they can grumble and stagnate, but they cannot fail. Failure is subjective and limited to a time and space measurement that will change relative to the reality in that moment.

Nursing has traversed some very difficult years and will no doubt continue to face challenges in this new millennium. We have found 10,000 ways that won't work: scarlet C. Let's gather the profession and design a way forward that empowers and strengthens nursing—let's create a vision, a mission, goals, and strategies that heal the profession of care and, in turn, close the chasms of care.

REVIEW QUESTIONS

1. What role do short-term goals play in a project?
2. Describe the impact management silos have on an organization.
3. List Kotter's eight stages of creating buy-in.
4. What are the risks of overcelebrating short-term goals?
5. What are the options when confronted with a roadblock?

REFERENCES

American Nurses Association (ANA). (2009). *About ANA*. Retrieved January 14, 2009, from http://www.nursingworld.org/FunctionalMenuCategories/AboutANA.aspx

Angelo, E. J. (2007). *Evidence based practice guidelines related to urinary catheterization*. Retrieved January 14, 2009, from http://www.acestar.uthscsa.edu/institute/su07/documents/3Angelo_000.pdf

Centers for Medicare & Medicaid Services (CMS). (2009a). *Deficit Reduction Act: Overview*. Retrieved May 19, 2009, from http://www.cms.hhs.gov/DeficitReductionAct

Centers for Medicare & Medicaid Services (CMS). (2009b). *Eliminating serious, preventable, and costly medical errors—never events*. Retrieved January 15, 2009, from http://www.cms.hhs.gov/apps/media/press/release.asp?Counter=1863

Gentile, M. C. (2008). The 21st century MBA. *strategy+business*. Retrieved June 24, 2009, from http://www.strategy-business.com/press/freearticle/08209

Gordon, S. (2005). *Nursing against the odds: How health care cost cutting, media stereotypes, and medical hubris undermine nursing and patient care*. Ithaca, NY: Cornell University Press.

International Council of Nursing (ICN). (2009). *ICN's vision for the future of nursing*. Retrieved January 15, 2009, from http://www.icn.ch/visionstatement.htm

Kotter, J. P. (1996). *Leading change*. Boston: Harvard Business School Press.

Liff, A. (2008). *Avoiding eight pitfalls of strategic planning*. Retrieved January 4, 2009, from http://www.allbusiness.com/print/601377-1=22eeq.html

National League for Nursing (NLN). (2009). *Mission and goals*. Retrieved May 19, 2009, from http://www.nln.org/aboutnln/ourmission.htm

Ohmae, K. (1988). Getting back to strategy. *Harvard Business Review*. Retrieved January 14, 2009, from http://hbr.harvardbusiness.org/1988/11/getting-back-to-strategy/ar/1

Trossman, S. (2008). BSN in ten. *American Nurse Today*, *3*(11). Retrieved May 21, 2009, from http://www.americannursetoday.com/Article.aspx?fid=5244&id=5272

Index